Artificial Intelligence and Machine Learning in 2D/3D Medical Image Processing

Artificial Intelligence and Machine Learning in 2D/3D Medical Image Processing

Edited by
Rohit Raja, Sandeep Kumar,
Shilpa Rani, and K. Ramya Laxmi

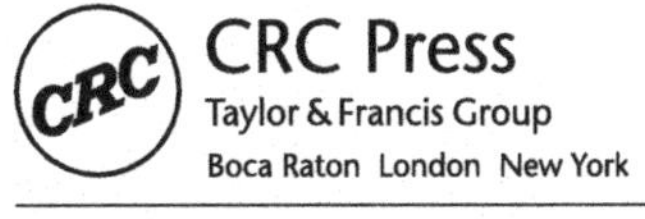

CRC Press is an imprint of the
Taylor & Francis Group, an informa business

First edition published 2021
by CRC Press
6000 Broken Sound Parkway NW, Suite 300, Boca Raton, FL 33487-2742

and by CRC Press
2 Park Square, Milton Park, Abingdon, Oxon, OX14 4RN

CRC Press is an imprint of Taylor & Francis Group, LLC

Library of Congress Cataloging-in-Publication Data

Names: Raja, Rohit, editor.
Title: Artificial intelligence and machine learning in 2D/3D medical image processing/ edited by Rohit Raja, Sandeep Kumar, Shilpa Rani, K. Ramya Laxmi.
Description: First edition. | Boca Raton: CRC Press, 2021. | Includes bibliographical references and index. | Summary: "Medical image fusion is a process which merges information from multiple images of the same scene. The fused image provides appended information that can be utilized for more precise localization of abnormalities. The use of medical image processing databases will help to create and develop more accurate and diagnostic tools'-- Provided by publisher.
Identifiers: LCCN 2020039590 (print) | LCCN 2020039591 (ebook) | ISBN 9780367374358 (hardback) | ISBN 9780429354526 (ebook)
Subjects: LCSH: Diagnostic imaging--Data processing. | Imaging systems in medicine.
Classification: LCC RC78.7.D53 .A78 2021 (print) | LCC RC78.7.D53 (ebook) | DDC 616.07/540285--dc23
LC record available at https://lccn.loc.gov/2020039590
LC ebook record available at https://lccn.loc.gov/2020039591

ISBN: 978-0-367-37435-8 (hbk)
ISBN: 978-0-429-35452-6 (ebk)

Typeset in Times New Roman
by MPS Limited, Dehradun

Contents

Preface

In this volume of Medical Image Processing, the study is concerned with interactions of all forms of radiation and tissue. The development of technology is used to extract clinically useful information from medical images. Medical Image fusion is a process which merges information from multiple images of the same setting and the resulting image retains the most valuable information and features of input images. Medical Image fusion can extend the range of operations, reduce uncertainties, and expand reliability. In the Medical Imaging field, different images exist of the same component of the same patient with dissimilar imaging devices, and the information provided by a variety of imaging modes is much adulatory each other's. The fused image provides appended information that can be utilized for more precise localization of abnormalities. Image Fusion is a process of combining the relevant information from a set of images into a single image, such that the resulting fused image will be more informative and consummate than any of the input images. Image fusion techniques can improve the quality and increase the application of these data. The most important applications of the fusion of images include medical imaging, tiny imaging, remote sensing, computer optics, and robotics. Feature of this book are

- The book highlights the framework of robust and novel methods for medical image processing techniques.
- Implementation strategies and future research directions meeting the design and application requirements of several modern and real time applications for long time.
- The book meets the current needs of the field. Advancement in Artificial Intelligence and Machine Learning in Medical Image processing are seldom reviewed in older books.
- Real Time Applications

We express our appreciation to all of the contributing authors who helped us tremendously with their contributions, time, critical thoughts, and suggestions to put together this peer-reviewed edited volume. The editors are also thankful to Apple Academic Press and their team members for the opportunity to publish this volume. Lastly, we thank our family members for their love, support, encouragement, and patience during the entire period of this work.

Rohit Raja
Sandeep Kumar
Shilpa Rani
K. Ramya Laxmi

Introduction

The main scope of this volume is to bring together concepts, methods and applications of medical image processing. The concept of the study is concerned with the interaction of all forms of radiation and tissue. The development of technology is used to extract clinically useful information from medical images. Medical Image Fusion is a process which merges information from multiple images of the same setting, and the resulting image retains the most valuable information and features of input images. Medical Image Fusion can extend the range of operations, reduce uncertainties and expand reliability. In the Medical Imaging field, different images exist of the same component of the same patient with dissimilar imaging devices, and the information provided by a variety of imaging modes is much adulatory each other's. The fused image provides appended information that can be utilized for more precise localization of abnormalities. Image Fusion is a process of combining the relevant information from a set of images into a single image such that the resulting fused image will be more informative and consummate than any of the input images alone. Image fusion techniques can improve the quality and increase the application of these data. The most important applications of the fusion of images include medical imaging, tiny imaging, remote sensing, computer optics, and robotics.

This book will target undergraduate graduate and postgraduate students, researchers, academicians, policy-makers, various government officials, academicians, technocrats, and industry research professionals who are currently working in the fields of academia research and the research industry to improve the quality of healthcare and life expectancy of the general public.

Chapter 1: This chapter introduces Biomedical Image processing, which has experienced dramatic growth and has been an fascinating area of interdisciplinary exploration, incorporating knowledge from mathematics, computer sciences, engineering, statistics, physics, biology, and medicine. Computer-aided analytical processing has already come to be a vital part of the scientific process. 3D imaging in medical study is the method used to acquire images of the body for scientific purpose in order to discover or study diseases. Worldwide, there are countless imaging strategies performed every week. 3D medical imaging is efficaciously growing because of developments in image processing strategies, including image recognition, investigation, and development. Image processing increases the proportion and extent of detected tissues. Currently, misperception has been produced among 2D and 3D machinery in health. This section presents the dissimilarity between these technologies and the software of both simple and complex image evaluation methods within the medical imaging discipline. This section also reviews how to demonstrate image interpretation challenges with the use of unique image processing systems, including division, arrangement, and registering strategies. Furthermore, it also discusses special kinds of medical imaging and modalities which contain CT test (pc tomography), MRI (scientific Resonance Imaging), Ultrasound, X-Ray, and so on. The important goals of this investigation are to provide a foundation for the creation of fundamental concepts and strategies for medical image processing and to encourage the pursuit of additional study and research in medical imaging processing. We will introduce the 3D Clinical Image Graph Processing and summarize related research depictions in this area and describe recent ultra-modern techniques. The software of 3D scientific imaging and 3D has been a success in offering answers to many complex scientific issues. As technology spreads, its applications continue to grow inside the industry.

Chapter 2: Epilepsy is a neurological afflictions which has affected around 1% of humanity. Epilepsy is generally recognized by the tendency of the cerebrum to generate abnormal electrical activity and other actions creating disturbances in the conventional working behavior of the mind. To gather information about the electrical activity of the human brain, EEG is the preferred option. In this research paper, we have proposed a novel deep Convolutional Neural Network model with back-propagation algorithms, wherein the model analyzes the signal to classify and segregate it into three unique classes namely pre-ictal, normal and seizure. The database employed for this study is the popular, publicly available benchmark Bonn University database. For analyzing the potential and how well the model has performed, we used sensitivity, specificity, and accuracy as the main performance metrics. Here, a 10-fold cross-validation technique was applied. The study resulted in an accuracy of 97.33%, sensitivity of 96.00% and specificity of 98%. The results were then analyzed with other existing work in this field.

Chapter 3: Digital image processing brought about a tremendous revolution in many fields, the medical field being one of them. Medical images are used to detect abnormalities and diseases in the human body; simply by analyzing them. During the acquisition process; noise signals may be introduced in these images, which will negatively impact the diagnostic process. Noise signals degrade the image quality by suppressing useful information present in the form of edges, fine structures, textures and so on. Hence, it is essential to suppress noise signals because noisy images may lead to false interpretations by radiologists. Suppression of noise signals from medical images is called "Medical Image De-noising". Some examples of medical images are Magnetic Resonance Images (MRI), Computed Tomography (CT) images, Ultra-Sound (US) images and so on. These images are corrupted by various noise signals. For example, MRI images are affected severely by noise, known as Rician noise; CT images are corrupted by Gaussian noise and US images are affected by multiplicative noise called speckle noise. To remove these unwanted noise signals, various filters have been proposed but none of these methods can be used as a global de-noising technique because any filter which can remove one noise effectively fails to remove others. Hence, it is necessary to develop a filter that can remove many noise signals because any image may be corrupted by more than one noise. This requirement motivates the researchers to achieve such a goal. In this chapter, a framework has been proposed to de-noise medical images, which reduces the effect of additive white Gaussian noise. It consists of various spatial domain filters, particularly the median filter and median modified Wiener filter. It also uses adaptive wavelet thresholding and total variation technique in parallel whose results are fused together using wavelet based fusion technique. This process is known as shrinkage combined enhanced total variation technique as it enhances the quality of de-noised images.

Chapter 4: In recent times, for the detection of nodules and lung segmentation, many Computer Aided Diagnosis systems have been designed to assist the radiologist. The two main factors which affect the accuracy and effectiveness of the detection of lung cancer are the nodule who has similar intensity and they are connected to a vessel and the nodule with typical weak edges, hence it is difficult to define the boundaries. In the present work the main objective is to handle the two above-mentioned problems with the use of a CADe system for segmentation and detection of nodule forms with CT Scan Images using LGXP method and Morphological Image processing. The advantage of using Local Gabor XOR Pattern (LGXP) and modified region growing algorithm for extensive feature set like texture contrast, correlation and shape are extracted. The present work has been analyzed using the data of different subjects of varying ages to reduce the number of errors and to decrease the time needed to examine the scan by a radiologist. There are five problems that can be associated with CADe for lung cancer detection: The first problem is the detection of noises and loss-less information in the CT image. Due to the presence of noise, the performance of the system may degrade. We have taken 10 CT scans or subjects from LIDC-IDRI, which include 5 different cases. The results found are highly satisfactory.

Chapter 5: Image fusion is a procedure which consolidates data from numerous images of a similar setting and the resulting images contain valuable highlights of information Images. Fusion of Images can broaden the scope of activity, diminish vulnerabilities and improve consistent quality. Currently in Medical Imaging fields, various image of a similar segment some portion of a similar patient with divergent symbolism gadgets, and the data gave by an assortment of imaging modes is a lot of adulatory one another. The melded Image gives added data that can be used for increasingly exact restriction of variations from the norm. This part concentrates on computerized Image Fusion and proposes a model for blending images, utilizing ANFIS, executes and look at execution. The proposed model is isolated into four sections: Read Image, Separate Image into shading channel (for RGB Images), Applying to ANFIS, and Combining shading channels.

Chapter 6: The advent of medical imaging has had a tremendous impact on the detection of various types of diseases. In this regard, medical image processing has made a large contribution in identifying numerous diseases, as well as reducing the human effort required in various healthcare applications. Currently, digital sensors are also used, along with standard image modalities such as Magnetic Resonance imaging (MRI), Compute Tomography (CT), ultrasound, X Rays. In the past, these diseases were examined by doctors or radiologists and thus were more prone to human error. In recent years, researchers have successfully used various image modalities for detecting and diagnosing the diseases. The various image modalities that are used to automate the process of detecting these diseases are described in this chapter. This chapter also emphasizes ecent advancements in the field of Medical Imaging, as well as describing future trends in the state-of-art image processing algorithms in providing efficient and affordable healthcare services.

Chapter 7: Diabetic Retinopathy is a major cause of peventable permanent blindness worldwide. To reduce the number of individuals suffering from this disease, annual screening must be performed on all diabetic patients. However, manual screening of all patients is not possible, as it requires greater numbers of medical personnel around the world. On the other hand, if adequate facilities are not made available, then there will be a steep increase in undiagnosed and untreated cases of Diabetic Retinopathy. Thus, a system is needed for automatic diagnosis of Diabetic Retinopathy. The system would refer cases with a high probablility of having the disease to the expert ophthalmologist. This system would be helpful in reducing the rate of eyesight loss and enable a proper and exact diagnosis. Here, an ensemble is proposed that classifies the images into normal and abnormal images. Ensemble consists of three different deep learning architectures. The ensemble's work and performance are computed using contrasting parameters and is found to be better than all the individual architectures.

Chapter 8: The examination and compression of clinical imagery is a significant area in Biomedical Engineering. The examintion of clinical images and data compression is a quickly developing field with emerging applications in health care services. Currently, digital techniques and applications in healthcare services are utilized for the diagnosis of patients. These techniques providing information about patients in the form of medical images require huge amounts of disk space to store the clinical information. Moreover, if any diagnostic center wanted to send this information to an expert for diagnostic purposes through a network, there is a requirement of larger bandwidth for the purpose of transmission. Therapeutic knowledge grows very rapidly and henceforth hospital requirements to accumulation vast amounts of patient information and data. Clinical images remain the most vital statistics about patients. Accordingly, diagnostic laboratories and hospitals have a massive quantity of patient images and data that require a corresponding massive storage space. More often, transmission bandwidth is inadequate to transmit all the pictures and data over an information channel. Thus, an image compression technique has been used to overcome these types of problems in the clinical field. In this paper, compression is performed with various kinds of wavelet functions to form a clinical picture and we propose the utmost fitting wavelet role which can achieve perfect reduction to a specified sort of clinical picture. For examine the routine of the wavelet role by means of the clinical pictures the loss of data amount is fixed. So that there is no information loss in the examination picture and determined their compression percentage in rate. The wavelet which provides utmost reduction in size of clinical picture with less loss of information has chosen for that image category.

Chapter 9: Alzheimer's Disease (AD) is one of the most common types of diseases amongst older adults and constitutes one the leading cause of death in senior citizens. To prevent Alzheimer's and provide early treatment, we have to accurately diagnosis Alzheimer's Disease and its prophase, which is called Mild Cognitive Impairment (MCI) in the healthcare sector. To recognize the type or stage of disease, it is essential to classify medical data and potentially develop a prediction model or system. The framework that we have developed consists of Machine Learning methods with PSO optimization and has been successfully applied to the classification of AD and Dementia. For the prediction of Alzheimer's Disease, we have used seven Machine Learning Algorithms such as Support Vector Machine Classification, Random Forest Classification, XgBoost Classifier, Decision Tree Classification, Adaboost Classifier, K-Neighbour Classifier, and Logistic Regression. Our best-proposed method is the Random Forest Classifier, which achieves the best accuracy of 85.71%.

Chapter 10: This chapter introduces Parkinson's syndrome, a dynamic condition of the central nervous system (CNS), affecting development & initiating shocks and solidness. It has five phases and influences more than millions of people each year throughout India. It is neuro-degenerative condition that influences the hormone known as dopamine creating neurons in the cerebrum. XGBoost is an additional Machine Learning calculation strategic considering velocity & implementation. XGBoost signifies extreme Gradient Boosting and depends upon a decision tree. In listed task,s we import XGB Classifier from xgboost library, which is a usage of scikit learn APIs for XGBoost arrangement. To assemble the model to precisely distinguish the onset of Parkinson's syndrome in individuals. In this Python AI venture, utilizing the Python libraries scikit learn, xgboost, pandas and NumPy, we assemble models utilizing a XGB Classifier. We'll stack the information, obtain the highlights and names, scale the highlights, at that point split the dataset, construct a XGB Classifier, and afterward ascertain the exactness of our model.

Chapter 11: Speech impairment is a technique in which speech sound signals are produced that are effective to communicate with others. Speech impairments can be any type; from mild impairment such as in occasionally struggling over a few words, to severe impairment, such as not being capable of producing speech sounds signals at all. The basic outcome is to study the hybrid model of machine learning for speech impairment. For effective machine learning results, it uses a specific model, effective techniques, knowledge parameters and advanced tree algorithms for displaying the valuable results. We rely on speech as one of the primary methods of communicating with others. Speech impairments in childhood can have a negative influence on social development. Speech impairments at all stages of life can lead to embarrassment and shame. The result of learning patterns on various human affliction diagnoses supports established medical specialists on the effects of starting treatment early, even though some results exhibit the same factors. In this paper, Parkinson's dataset from the UCI library is used with the top four speech-related parameters. It obtains a higher accuracy level with a hybrid model compared with the other classifiers.

Chapter 12: This chapter introduces the use of Machines and Computers in the medical field. Currently, machine learning, artificial intelligence, plays an important role in the medical field, as well in recent medical measures, the handling of patient knowledge, and medical background. This proposed article aims to provide a capable method to accurately predict the biopsy result. First, the authors applied different classifiers available in WEKA and prepared graphs for 10 different algorithms; namely Random Subspace, J48, SMO, Bagging, Simple Logistics, LWL, Multiclass Classifier Updateable, lbk, Naive Bayes, Naive Bayes Updateable. On the basis of the group, the Machine Learning mold of Simple Logistics was advanced. Practical outputs indicate that the advanced Simple Logistics machine learning model has improved results in comparison to ensemble-based machine learning methods. The proposed work describes a good method of performing bioassays on high-dimensional balanced data.

Chapter 13: This chapter looks at the Lung, the most important organ in our cellular respiration system and which is situated in the chest cavity. Lungs are a set of spongy organs which allow us to breathe properly. Lungs are responsible for providing oxygen to the human body and sending carbon dioxide out of the body. The exchange of these gases is called respiration. In contemporary life lung cancer is a common disease and the cause of a greater number of deaths around the world. Lung cancer is the most deadly cancer other than breast cancer, bone cancer and so on. The primary cause of lung cancer is smoking. Although nonsmokers can also get lung cancer, the rate is ten times less than it is for the person who smokes. Diagnosing the lung tumor in the early stages is a very difficult task but if detected in the last stage, the only treatment option is to remove the cancerous lung. Therefore, early detection is vital.

Editors

Rohit Raja is working as associate professor in the IT Department at the Guru Ghasidas, Vishwavidyalaya, Bilaspur (CG). He has done PhD in Computer Science and Engineering in 2016 from C. V. Raman University, India. His primary research interests include face recognition, signal processing and networking and data mining. He has successfully filed 10 patents. He has 80 research publications to his credit in various international/national journals (including IEEE, Springer etc.) and in proceedings of reputed international/national conferences (including Springer and IEEE). He was invited thrice as a guest in Scopus indexed IEEE/Springer conferences. He has been invited four times, being an expert, in various colleges and universities in India. He has the following awards to his credit: “Excellence in Research” Award under the category of HEI Professor by Auropath Global Awards, 2019; the “Distinguished Research Award”, I2OR Awards 2019, during the 4th International Conclave on Interdisciplinary Research for Sustainable Development 2020 (IRSD 2020); and the second runner up award in grand finale of Smart India Hackathon, 2017, Ministry of Skill Development and Entrepreneurship, Government of India.

He is a member of professional international society including IEEE, ISTE, CSI, ACM etc. He is editor/reviewer of many peer-reviewed and refereed journals (including IEEE, Springer, enderscience).

Sandeep Kumar is presently working as a professor in the Department of Electronics & Communication Engineering, Sreyas Institute of Engineering & Technology, Hyderabad, India. He has good academic and research experience in various areas of electronics and communication. His areas of research include embedded system, image processing, biometrics and machine learning. He has successfully filed eight patents – seven national and one international. He was invited thrice as a guest in Scopus indexed IEEE/Springer conferences. He has been invited four times, being an expert, in various colleges and universities in India. He has published 70 research papers in various international/national journals (including IEEE, Springer etc.) and in the proceedings of the reputed international/national conferences (including Springer and IEEE). He has been awarded the “Best Paper Presentation” award in Nepal and in India, respectively, 2017 and 2018. He has been awarded the “Best Performer Award” in Hyderabad, India, 2018. He has also been awarded the “Young Researcher Award” in Thailand, 2018, and the “Best Excellence Award” in Delhi, 2019. He is an active member of 17 professional international societies. He has been nominated in the board of editors/reviewers of 25 peer-reviewed and refereed journals (including IEEE and Springer). He has conducted three international conferences and six workshops. He is also attended 24 seminars, workshops and short-term courses in IITs etc. He is a research guide for a number of Ph.D and M.Tech students.

Shilpa Rani is presently working as an assistant professor in the Department of Computer Science and Engineering, Neil Gogte Institute of Technology, Hyderabad, India. She has good academic and research experience in various areas of computer science. Her area of research includes image processing, IOT, and big data. She has successfully filed three patents. She has published a number of research papers in various international/national journals (including IEEE, Springer etc.). She has been awarded the gold medal in 2012 during M.Tech. She is an active member of 10 professional international societies. She has been nominated in the board of editors/reviewers of four peer-reviewed and refereed journals. She has also attended 15 seminars, workshops and short-term courses in JNTUH and others. She has published two text books *Logical & Functional Programming*, Ashirwad Publication, 2009–2010 and *Software Engineering*, VAYU Education of India, 2011. Her third book has been accepted at an international level by Taylor & Francis, USA

K. Ramya Laxmi has worked as team lead and senior software developer at InfoTech Pvt Ltd for four years. Presently she is working as associate professor in the CSE Department at the Sreyas Institute of Engineering and Technology, Hyderabad. Her research interests cover the fields of data mining, machine learning and image processing. She has good academics and research experience in various areas of Computer Science. She has good hands-on-experience in PHP and Python and has knowledge of tools such as Pentaho and Weka, and is apt at analysing statistics using R-Programming.

Contributors

Renuka Arora
Guru Kashi University
Bathinda, India

Vineet Awasthi
Department of Information Technology
Dr. C. V. Raman University
Bilaspur, India

Rohit Bajaj
Chandigarh University
India

Devanand Bhonsle
Sstc
Bhilai, India

Vivek Kumar Chandra
Csit Drug
India

Vaishali Devi
Govt. College
Alewa, India

Saurabh Dewangan
Nit
Raipur, India

D. Ghai
Lovely Professional University
Phagwara, India

Akanksha Gupta
It Department
Ggv Central University
Bilaspur, India

Rahul Hooda
Govt. College
Alewa, India

Swati Jain
Govt. J. Y. Chhattisgarh College
Raipur, India

Rekh Ram Janghel
Nit
Raipur, India

Maguluri Sudeep Joel
Sreyas Institute of Engineering and Technology
Hyderabad, India

Dinesh Kumar
Guru Kashi University
India

Munish Kumar
Eiepl
Delhi, India

Prashant Kumar
Nit
Raipur, India

Sandeep Kumar
ECE Department
Sreyas Institute of Engineering and Technology
Hyderabad, India

K. Ramya Laxmi
CSE Department
SIET
Hyderabad, India

Kamal Mehta
Computer Science and Information Technology
Mukesh Patel School of Technology and Management
Nmims Shirpur, India

Rohit Miri
Department of Information Technology
Dr. C. V. Raman University
Bilaspur, India

Pankaj Kumar Mishra
Rcet
Bhilai Durg, India

Saroj Kumar Pandey
Nit
Raipur, India

Raj Kumar Patra
Cse Department
Cmr Technical Campus
Hyderabad, India

Lokesh Pawar
Chandigarh University
India

Rohit Raja
Department of IT
Ggv Central University
Bilaspur, India

Shilpa Rani
CSE Department
NGIT
Hyderabad, India

K. Rawal
Lovely Professional University
Phagwara, India

G. Sethi
Lovely Professional University
Phagwara, India

Anuj Kumar Sharma
BRCMCET
MD University
India

Prakash C. Sharma
Department of Information Technology
Manipal University
Jaipur, India

G. R. Sinha
Mit
Mandley, Myanmar

Upasana Sinha
J. K. Institute of Engineering
Bilaspur, India

Laxmikant Tiwari
Department of Csit
Dr. C. V. Raman University
Bilaspur, India

Kshitiz Varma
Csvtu
Bhilai Durg, India

Archana Verma
Nit
Raipur, India

1 An Introduction to Medical Image Analysis in 3D

Upasana Sinha, Kamal Mehta, and Prakash C. Sharma

CONTENTS

1.1 INTRODUCTION

3D Image Analysis is the visualization, processing and evaluation of 3D photo statistics through geometric transformation, filtering, picture segmentation and other morphological operations. 3D conception forms the basis of contemporary radiology. 3D experimental imaging is a modern visual imaging scientific expertise that affords an enriched image of the interior body for scientific assessment making use of 3D imaging modalities. 3D scientific imaging provides more effective pictures of blood vessels and better images of bones. It is undisputable that 3 Dimensional (3D) imaging is continuously improving with the continued enhancement of instrumentation.

1.2 COMPARISON BETWEEN 2D AND 3D TECHNIQUES IN MEDICAL IMAGING

2D and 3D refer to the genuine dimensions in a computer workspace. 2D is "flat"; using horizontal and vertical (X and Y) dimensions; the image graph has solely two dimensions and turns into a line. 3D provides the depth (Z) dimension. This 0.33-

dimension permits rotation and visualization from a couple of perspectives. It is in effect the distinction between an image and a sculpture.

For example, taking the pattern image graphs of echocardiography, there is the volumetric method to statistics acquisition in 2D and 3D (Figure 1.1).

Medical imaging has developed extensively since the early days of CT scanners and mammography equipment. With 3D scientific imaging, healthcare professionals were able to obtain access to fresh angles, resolutions, and small detail that provided an outstanding portrait of the physical section in query, at the same time as reducing the amount of radioactivity in patients [1, 2, 3]. In recent decades, the quantity of 3D scientific imaging has doubled in number every month to about one hundred thirty instances per day by 2018. The science of scanning has become a superior technology in creating statistical units that can make 3D images clearer with greater decision precision and much less noise and artifacts. Medical imaging has superior technological know-how in particular when it comes to these slice counts; it permits us to enlarge the precision of the pictures that we are shooting and, additionally signify the 3d mannequin of the anatomy, which used to be a substitute no longer feasible in the early days of the process (Figure 1.2).

1.3 IMPORTANCE OF 3D MEDICAL IMAGE

As we are all aware, medical imaging encompasses distinctive imaging modalities (a kind of technology used to gather structural or purposeful pictures of the body) such as radiography, ultrasound, nuclear prescription, computed tomography (CT), magnetic resonance and seen light. This requires techniques to image graph the body for diagnostictic and therapeutic purpose and performs an essential function in enhancing medical treatment. This proves that clinical imaging is regularly justified in the follow up of an ailment already recognized or treated [4, 5].

Medical imaging, in particular X-ray, primarily built investigations plus ultrasonography, stays necessary for a range of scientific putting and by altogether predominant stages of fitness precaution. In communal fitness and protective remedy by way of suitable as in each healing and relaxing care, good choices rely on the right analyses. However, medicinal/scientific decisions might also

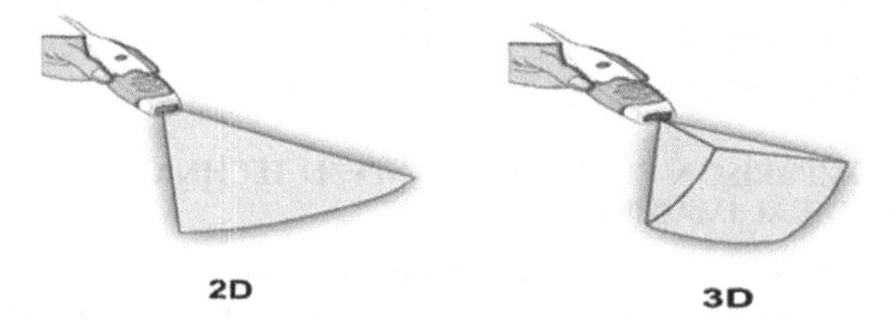

FIGURE 1.1 2D (left panel) and 3D (right panel) Echocardiography Visualization Image.

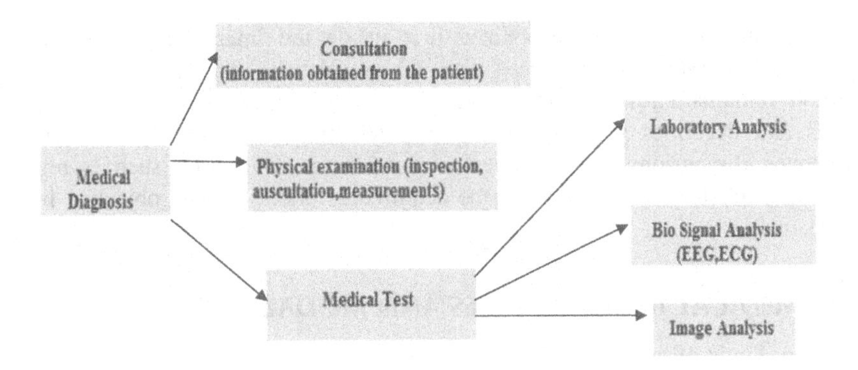

FIGURE 1.2 Medical Imaging.

remain adequate former to therapy of numerous circumstances, the practise of diagnostic imaging offerings is dominant in confirming, efficiently measuring and authenticating publications of several ailments as nicely as in an evaluating reaction to treatment. Through accelerated health care coverage plus the growing accessibility of clinical apparatus, the range of world imaging-based strategies continues to grow significantly. Accurate and safe forms of imaging remain necessary in clinical practice and can reduce the use of pointless procedures. For instance, some medical interventions can be prevented if easy diagnostic imaging such as ultrasound is available.

It is well known that 3D picture processing is a tremendous tool for extent calculation, measurement, and quantitative analysis. It starts off evolved from 3D fashions of the patient, routinely recognized and extracted from anatomical structures, analysis, and surgical simulations can be supported. Moreover, with the usage of augmented actuality capabilities, it is feasible to merge preoperative or intraoperative information with reality, which is a precious device in the discipline of image guided surgery. 3D technological know-how has changed scientific imaging developing the opportunity for talent mapping with excessive decision microscopy. It has the capacity to discover character neurons, hint connections between them, and visualize organelles' internal neurons.

The fundamental and first step in 3D image processing is the division of a picture which organizes pixels into substances or collections. 3D image division makes it practical to make 3D versions for more than one object and function with quantitative evaluation aimed at the extent, mass, and different factors of identified substances.

New images are taken, whether by CT, MRI, or microscopy image diagram as a 3D range of voxels/pixels. Individual voxel takes a greyscale vary from 0 to 65535 in the sixteen-bit pixel instance or 0 to 255 in the eight-bit pixel case. A segmented image, on the different hand, provides a less complicated explanation of substances that allows an introduction of 3D level methods or shows point data. When the fresh image graph is conveniently displayed as 3D evaluation, then imagining requires clearly described objective limits after growing models. Taking as an instance, to generate a 3D version of humanoid intelligence from an MRI image, the intelligence wishes to be recognized first inside the image graph and before its periphery manifest and used for 3D translation. The pixel recognition method remains known as image division, which recognises the qualities of pixels and describes the limitations for pixels that go to an identical group. Moreover, dimensions and numerical evaluation for restrictions such as region, boundary, quantity, and extent can be acquired effortlessly once objective limits are distinct.

1.4 MEDICAL IMAGING TYPES AND MODALITIES

Different kinds of medicinal imaging contain:

i. **CT (Computed Tomography)**
CT or CAT (pc axial tomography) images are the shape of X-ray that generates 3D images for analysis. It makes use of X-rays towards frame supply section images. A scanner with CT takes an outsized round establishing aimed at the affected person lying on a motorized desk. The X-ray delivers in addition a sensor then it rotates around the affected idividual, generating a slight 'fan-shaped' ray of X-rays that permits via part of the patient's physique to make a picture. Those pictures are then assembled into single, or multiple images of interior organs and tissues. The CT scans supply higher transparency in comparison to traditional X-rays through greater unique picture graphs of the internal organs, bones, mild tissues, and blood vessels within the frame. The advantages of the use of CT scans outweigh the risks, which similar to X-rays, include cancer, damage to an unborn child, or allergic reaction to the chemicals in contrast material. In many instances, using a CT scan removes the need for experimental surgical operations. It is essential that when scanning children, the radiation dosage is lower than that used for adults. In many hospitals, a paediatrics CT scanner is available for that purpose.

ii. **MRI (Magnetic Resonance Imaging)**
MRI scans generate diagnostic image graphs without emission of dangerous radiation. Magnetic resonance Imaging (MRI) makes use of strong magnetic placed besides radio waves to produce pictures of the body which cannot be detected by X-rays or CT scans, i.e., it enables joints, ligaments and soft tissue to be visible [6, 7, 8]. The MRI is frequently used to observe interior detail to detect strokes, tumours, spinal cord accidents, aneurysms, and intelligence function. We realize the majority of the human body consists of water, and every water molecule consists of a hydrogen nucleus (proton) which become allied in a magnetic field. An MRI scanner provides a secure magnetic field to support the proton 'spins'. A radio frequency is then applied which propels the protons to 'flip' their spins in advance than return to their proper arrangement. Protons in particular body organs revert to their regular spins at dissimilar rates so the MRI can differentiate among numerous types of tissue and detect any deformities. In what way the molecules 'flip' then arrive back at

their ordinary spin arrangements is noted and processed into a picture. MRI doesn't use ionizing radiation and is gradually being cast-off at some stage in pregnancy and not using a thing results at the unborn infant mentioned. But there are dangers related to using MRI scanning, and it isn't endorsed as a primary analysis.Due to the strong magnets used, it is not suitable for individuals with any kind of steel implant, synthetic joints, and so on because of the chance they might be dislodged or heated up in the magnetic field.

iii. **ULTRASOUND**

Ultrasound remains the most secure method of scientific imaging and takes a large variety of packages. There aren't any risk to the use of ultrasound, and it remains one of the best low-cost types of medical imaging available to us. Ultrasound makes use of sound waves instead of ionizing emission. High-frequency sound waves travel through the body with the aid of a transducer. Those waves then bounce back once they hit denser surfaces in the body and that is used to generate an image for prognosis. Another type of ultrasound often used is the 'Doppler' – an extraordinary method of the use of sound waves that allows the bloodflow via arteries and veins to be visible. Due to the absence of risk in ultrasound, it is the first choice of imaging in pregnancy. However, because its uses are considerable – emergency prognosis, cardiac, spine, and internal organs – it often is the first imaging option for patients.

iv. **X-ray**

X-ray imaging – X-ray consitutes the oldest and most used form of imaging; indeed, most people have had at least one X-ray in their life. In 1895, it was discovered that X-rays are a form of electromagnetic radiation. X-rays work on a wavelength and frequency that we are not able to view with the bare human eye, but it can penetrate through the pores and skin to create an image of what's underneath. Generally used for detecting skeletal problems, X-rays can be used to detect cancers through mammography and digestive troubles through barium swallows and enemas. X-rays can be used extensively use as they are low cost, rapid, and effortless for the affected person to bear. But there are risks related to the use of radioactivity for X-ray imaging. In all instances, the affected individual who has an X-ray receives a dose of radiation. The exposure is brief, but there is a slight risk of radiation-precipitated cancers or cataracts later in life or harm to an embryo or foetus in a pregnant woman. Most of the dangers are moderated through using X-rays where strictly necessary and properly safeguarding the rest of the body with a protective shield.

1.5 COMPUTER VISION SYSTEM WORKS IN 3D IMAGE ANALYSIS

The corporation of the laptop vision tool is noticeably application based. There are capabilities that are discovered in many computer imaginative and prescient structures (Figure 1.3).

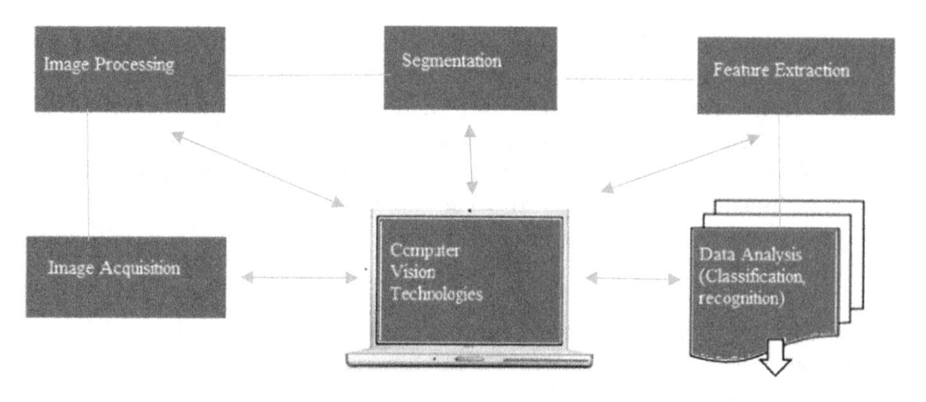

FIGURE 1.3 Computer Vision System.

- **Image Acquisition**
- **Pre-processing**
- **Feature Extraction** — **Image Processing**
- **Detection/Segmentation**
- **High level processing**
- **Decision Making**

Image Acquisition: It is a system of transforming the analogy global round us into double records collected of 0'S and 1'S, inferred as virtual images; e.g., client 3D cameras & laser range detectors.

Image Processing: Image acquisition is considered to be first step of image processing and second step in computer imaginative and perceptive. Procedures are utilized for binary statistics obtained in the primary stage to deduce low-level records on additives of the image graph. For example, the sort of statistic remains categorised by using picture ends, aspect sides, or sections. They are the primary geometric element that assembles substances in snapshots. They constitute the best geometric factors that assemble substances in images.

This 2nd step generally includes superior carried out arithmetic algorithms and strategies.

Low level image processing algorithm includes:

i. Edge detection. This is a hard and fast mathematical technique with the goal of identifying factors in a virtual photograph in which the photo brightness changes sharply or, more officially, has discontinuities. The factors at which image brightness changes are usually prepared into a set of curved line segments termed edges [9]. It is one of the vital steps in image processing, picture evaluation, and a computer imaginative and prescient approach.

Segmentation: Our primary effort is to extend the correctness of segmentation. The early stage consists of utilizing a number of filters (imply, Gaussian blur, region detection) and bit operations similar to histogram equalization and standardisation [10, 11]. These actions also need to be utilized in each photograph one at a time, or there are versions of these systems in 3D. An act in 3D is characterized by means of the use of a chain of 2d pictures (slices) organized in a row. Three coordinates each have a voxel. The initial two coordinates, x, and y characterize one pixel on a slice and the 0.33 one, z, represents the order of slice. At primary, the 3D image graph is geared up for segmentation. The aim of this method is to break up the image graph into continuous factors. Those components can be overlapping and collectively can cover the entire picture. Capabilities are calculated for each such segment.

Medical image graph: Division is the technique of automatic or semi-computerized recognition of interior boundaries a second before the 3D image. The crucial state of clinical picture division is the excessive inconsistency in the medical image. The analysis of the situation shows the maximum modes of the variant. Moreover, numerous special modalities (X-ray, CT, MRI, microscopy, pet, SPECT, Endoscopy, OCT, and plenty of greater) stay castoff towards generating medical images. An anticipated final outcome of the segmentation can now be used to build up similarly to diagnostic insights. Feasible purposes remain the computerized dimensions of organs, mobile telephone counting, or simulations established totally on the removed edge records.

Classification: Probably image graph remains the most essential segment in digital picture evaluation [10]. It is the primary class to have a "pretty image" or a picture, showing the importance of shades illustrating a number of factors of the basic terrain. However, this is ineffective until it is understood what the descriptions suggest. (PCI, 1997). Primary type strategies are supervised classification and unsupervised type.

By supervised type, we recognise instances of the material modules (i.e., land cowl type) of the hobby within the image and are referred to as "training websites" (Figure 1.4). The image graph handling software application tool is then used to strengthen a statistical description of the reflectance for each reality magnificence. This level is often termed as "signature evaluation" and can additionally include creating a description as clean as they mean or the vogue of reflectance on each band, or as complex as special analyses of the imply modifications and covariance over all bands. As soon as a statistical representation has been finished for every report class, the picture is then categorized with the means of analysing the reflectance for each pixel and creating a preference around which of the initials it most resembles. (Eastman, 1995)

Unsupervised type is a technique that inspects a big range of unidentified pixels and splits into a wide sort of class primarily founded mostly on herbal groupings current day in the picture values. In the evaluation of supervised classification, the unsupervised class no longer requires analyst-targeted coaching facts. The easy statement remains that value inner a assumed cover kind ought to be shut collected inside the dimension vicinity (i.e., Have comparable grey levels), whereas information in one in all a kind commands need to be relatively properly separated (i.e., Have very precise grey ranges) (PCI, 1997; Lillesand and Kiefer, 1994; Eastman, 1995). The programmes that cease end outcome from the unsupervised category are spectral ranked which primarily built on herbal alliances of the image

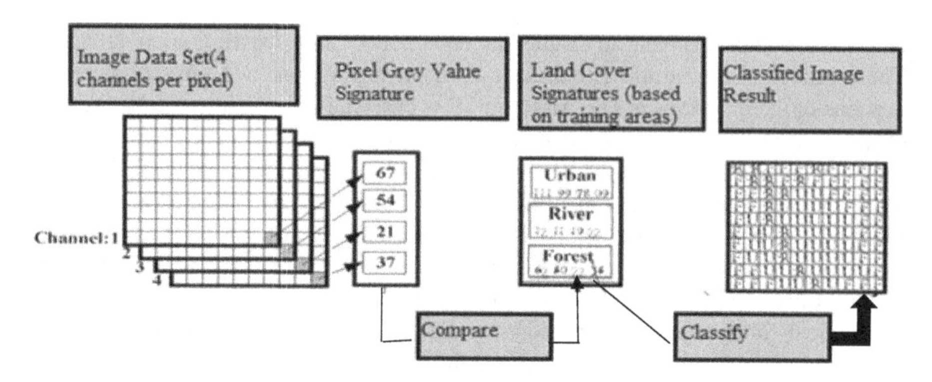

FIGURE 1.4 Steps in Supervised Classification.

graph values, the uniqueness of the spectral category will not be known in the beginning and one will have to compare categorised statistics to some shape of reference information (including large scale imagery, maps, or internet site online visits) to decide the identification and informational values of the spectral training. Consequently, within the supervised approach, to define useful statistics instructions and then take a look at their spectral reparability; inside the unsupervised method, the computer defines a spectrally separable class, and then describe their statistics price. (PCI, 1997; Lillesand and Kiefer, 1994).

Unsupervised type is becoming more well-known in groups involved in prolonged-time period GIS database upkeep. The motive is that there are actually structures that use grouping methods which are surprisingly short and minute within the nature of operational parameters [10]. Therefore, it is possible to train GIS assessment with only a familiarity with far-flung detecting to undertake classifications that meet regular map accuracy standards. With appropriate ground reality accuracy evaluation tactics, this device can grant a remarkably rapid capability of producing quality land cover facts on a continuing foundation.

High Level Pre-processing: The final phase of the computer image process is the investigation of the records, which will permit the building of results. High-level algorithms are functional, by means of exchanging the image data and the low-level data computed in earlier steps (Figure 1.5).

Examples of high-level image analysis are:

1. 3D scene mapping
2. Object recognition
3. Object tracking

1.6 VARIOUS TECHNIQUES IN 3D IMAGE PROCESSING IN MEDICAL IMAGING

There are many techniques one could use whilst processing 3D image records. Those strategies range based on the tasks to be accomplished– together with importing, visualizing, processing, and analysing the statistics.

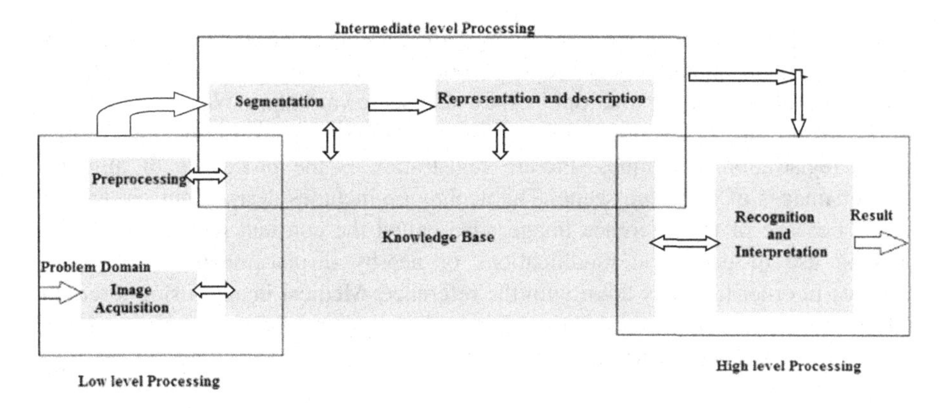

FIGURE 1.5 Levels of Pre-processing.

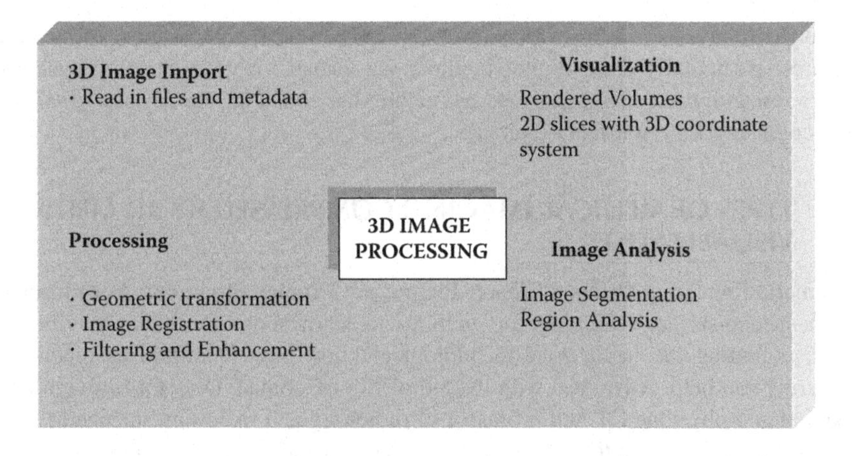

FIGURE 1.6 Key Components of a 3D Image Processing Workflow.

3D picture processing is generally utilized in medical imaging to read DICOM or NIfTI pictures from radiographic resources like MRI or CT scans. One may also use 3D image graph processing strategies in microscopy to detect and examine tissue samples or hint neurons (Figure 1.6).

Image Import and Visualization: 3D image information can originate from a range of tools and document layouts. To successfully import and visualize 3D images, it is vital to obtain access to the underlying data and metadata for the images. One could imagine 3D images using a range of strategies depending on the facts needed to be examined. In a few programs, one could imagine the 3D statistics as a reduced quantity.

Image Filtering and Enhancement: 3D images generally include undesirable noise that confuses or deemphasizes the purposes of the sizes that one is involved in. Making use of image filters, normalizing image evaluation, or performing morphological operations are not unusual methods for doing away with noise after 3D images.

Image Registration: While functioning with datasets of 3D pictures, the images are generally occupied from one kind of tool, or as a device is moving, that could present misalignment via rotation, or skew and scale variations. We are able to put off or lessen this misalignment by the use of 3D geometric variations and image graph registration techniques. Picture registration is the procedure of aligning greater images of the same scene. This technique includes designating one image graph because of the reference image, also called the constant image graph, and making use of geometric modifications or nearby displacements to the other pictures in order that they align with the reference. Medical image fusion refers to the fusion of medical pictures obtained from different modalities. Scientific picture fusion enables medical analysis through a manner of improving the first class of the pictures.

Filtering and Enhancement: We will lessen noise or beautify pictures by the use of image graph filtering methods like Gaussian filtering, box filtering, or picture morphology.

Image Analysis: Picture evaluation is the extraction of significant records from pictures; particularly from digital pictures via virtual image processing systems. Image research tasks may be as easy as reading bar coded tags or as state-of-the-art as recognising a person from their face.

1.7 TYPES OF MEDICAL IMAGING COMPRESSED BY 3D MEDICAL VISUALIZATION

Cinematic Rendering Offers a Clearer Picture of Complex Structures: For instance, when specialists are searching for methods to learn about complex areas of the body, including the heart, new technological know-how identified as cinematic rendering can help. Advanced with the aid of Eliot Fishman, Director of diagnostic imaging and physique CT and professor of radiology and radiology science at John Hopkins medicines, the technological information yields realistic pictures from the unification of 3D CT or 3D MRI scans by volumetric conception by way of distinct computer-generated image knowledge. This technique helps physicians whilst diagnosing illness, supervising surgical treatment, and planning a course of action. Cinematic rendering allows healthcare specialists to understand masses extra of the texture of the analysis (Figure 1.7).

Related to how ray locating makes someone's pores and skin appear larger and permeable within the films, cinematic rendering offers a detailed appearance of the texture of tumours, which allows the delivery of extra data for medical doctors to determine whether or not or not or no longer is a tumour cancerous. "With these textures, the greater precisely we can render and visualize them as people—the texture of the anatomy or the tumor—I assume the richer the statistics for medical doctors to interpret," Powell says.

Tomosynthesis Recovers Breast Cancer Recognition: Breast imaging has evolved from 2D mammography to 3D chemosynthesis (from time to time known as 3D mammography), which allows radiologists to capture images at numerous perspectives and show tissues on numerous depths at a greater level than would be

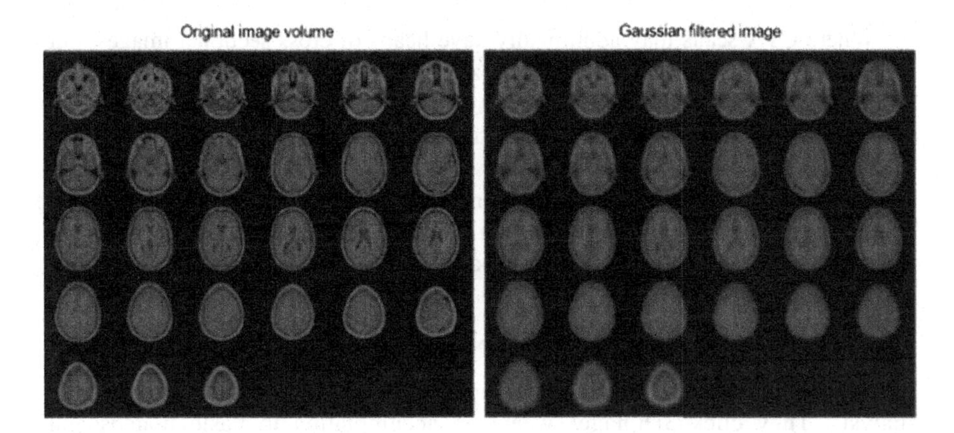

FIGURE 1.7 MRI Images of a Human Brain Using 3D Gaussian Filtering.

possible with a set of pictures only. This technique could permit radiologists to view images in 3D in a much more realistic manner, as noted by Harris.

"Tomosynthesis has been proven to enhance the care for breast most cancers detection and is extra sensitive, especially in sufferers at excessive danger or with dense breasts," Harris explains. "It helps to differentiate matters that may be misinterpreted that are probably different artifacts.

Artificial Intelligence Takes Medical Imaging to the Next Level: The last five years have brought about massive advancements in imaging, due to the powerful mixture of talent and 3D clinical imaging. At the GPU technology conference in March 2018, Nvidia introduced mission Clara, a "digital scientific AI supercomputer" that uses enhanced calculating competence than may be done with 3D volumetric rendering, in keeping with the work of Powell.

"AI should inject efficiency into clinical imaging, in particular when it comes to detecting organs or anomalies. For example, via combining photograph visualization and AI, cardiologists can measure ejection fraction—the share of blood pumped thru the coronary heart every time it contracts—in a lots shorter length of time barring having to kind via big statistics units and observe the anatomy via sight."

Usually, cardiologists and radiologists have the practice so that they really theoretically capture what's happening, but AI is in a position to deliver a correct, tough-number dimension to truly extending the opportunities that the analysis is as proper as it is able to be, Powell says [1, 12, 13].

3D Computing Tomography Angiography Maps Vascular Anomalies: At Massachusetts General Hospital, Harris researches 3D computed tomography angiography (CTA), in which medical experts can imagine arterial and venous vessels by way of a CT method. Professionals like Harris and his team practise CTA to record stenosis, aneurysms, dissections, and extraordinary vascular anomalies. On the side of 3D imaging, scientific experts can get an improved experience of what they're observing in analysis and pathology, as well as any potential artifacts.

"Where CTA scans may additionally have heaps of cross-sectional images, our 3D technologists can succinctly summarize a small set of 3D pics for the case so radiologists and referring medical doctors can examine it effectively barring having to do all the processing themselves," Harris says.

Additionally, despite the fact that MRIs and CT scans begin as second, they may be converted into 3D via management in 3D software, Harris explains. "It's no longer 3D through default, however you can take a stack of 2D facts units and manipulate it in 3D in a range of one-of-a-kind ways," he says.

1.8 3D ULTRASOUND SHORTENS THE IMAGING DEVELOPMENT

By 3D ultrasound, extremely-sonographers analysis to inspect a patient's analysis. They click 3Dimage sweeps in accumulation to basic images and deliver the pictures to a 3D computer. A 3D ultrasound technician then evaluations the pix and generates more 3D perspectives earlier than they go to the radiologist.

"The technologist will see whether or not the sonographer has captured the whole anatomy with the scan, if there may be negative photograph satisfactory or if they have ignored anything," Harris says. "They can have the ultra-sonographer replace the scan if necessary."

In 2003, Harris and his group started the usage of an attachment for the probe that takes a "smooth sweep of the anatomy" and reconstructs the data as a 3D records set. "If there is something in the snapshots they do not see clearly, we can reconstruct extra views from the uncooked information besides having to name the affected person back," Harris says. Now not only does this technique beautify efficiency for radiologists, ultrasonography, and patients, it also inserts elasticity into the method; as ultrasound tests can nowadays be received through satellite TV with computer imaging locations.

1.9 CONCLUSION

Basically, this chapter concludes that 3D imaging permits customers to replicate and analyse parts and objects in full 3D shape. This opens up limitless possibilities for first-rate manipulative measures and allow for an incredible outlet for visualizing the object in digital form. The most common benefits 3D imaging offer consist of non-negative 3D imaging strategies; it can provide fast and accurate results, the supply for giant analysis, to make certain element consistency and reliability and to permit attitude on excellent manipulate.

REFERENCES

1. Yong Yang, Shuying Huang, Nini Rao, "Medical Image Fusion via an Effective Wavelet-Based Approach", *Journal on Advances in Signal Processing*, 2010.
2. Rani Anju, Gagandeep Kaur, "Image Enhancement Using Image Fusion Techniques", IJARSSE, September 2014.

3. A. P. James, B. V. Dasarathy, "Medical Image Fusion: A Survey of the State of the Art", Information Fusion, 2014.
4. Shraddha Shukla, Rohit Raja, "A Survey on Fusion of Color Images", *International Journal of Advanced Research in Computer Engineering & Technology (IJARCET)*, Volume 5, Issue 6, June 2016.
5. Shraddha Shukla, Rohit Raja, "Digital Image Fusion using Adaptive Neuro-Fuzzy Inference System", *International Journal of New Technology and Research (IJNTR)*, Volume 2, Issue 5, May 2016, pp. 101–104.
6. Keshika Jangde, Rohit Raja, "Study of an Image Compression Based on Adaptive Direction Lifting Wavelet Transform Technique", *International Journal of Advanced and Innovative Research (IJAIR)*, Volume 2, Issue 8, 2013, pp. 2278–7844.
7. Keshika Jangde, Rohit Raja, "Image Compression Based on Discrete Wavelet and Lifting Wavelet Transform Technique", *International Journal of Science, Engineering and Technology Research (IJSETR)*, Volume 3, Issue 3, 2014, pp. 394–399.
8. Yamini Chouhan, Rohit Raja, "Robust Face Recognition snd Pose Estimation System", *International Journal of Science, Engineering and Technology Research (IJSETR)*, Paper ID: IJSETR-2474, Volume 3, Issue 1, 2014.
9. A. Kaur, Amrit Kaur, "Comparison of Mamdani-Type and Sugeno-Type Fuzzy Inference Systems for Air Conditioning System", IJSCE, Volume 2, Issue 2, May 2012.
10. Jionghua Teng, Suhuan Wang, Jingzhou Zhang, Xue Wang, "Algorithm of Medical Images Based on Fuzzy Logic", Seventh International Conference on Fuzzy Systems and Knowledge Discovery (FSKD 2010) "Fusion", 2010.
11. Pratibha Sharma, Manoj Diwakar, Sangam Choudhary, "Application of Edge Detection for Brain Tumor Detection", *International Journal of Advanced Research in Electronics and Communication Engineering (IJARECE)*", Volume 4, Issue 6, June 2015.
12. J. P. W. Pluim, J. B. A. Maintz, M. A. Viergever, "Mutual-information-based Processing of Medical Images: A Survey", *IEEE Transactions on Medical Imaging*, Volume 22, Issue 8, 2013.
13. C. C. Benson, V. L. Lajish, Kumar Rajamani "Brain Tumor Extraction from MRI Brains Images using Marker Based Watershed Algorithm" 3189 78-1-4799-8792-4/15/ $31.00 c 2015 IEEE.

2 Automated Epilepsy Seizure Detection from EEG Signals Using Deep CNN Model

Saroj Kumar Pandey, Rekh Ram Janghel, Archana Verma, Kshitiz Varma, and Pankaj Kumar Mishra

CONTENTS

2.1 INTRODUCTION

Roughly 50 million people are suffering from epilepsy globally, according to the study by the WHO (World Health Organization) in 2017 [1]. Approximately 10% of people are affected with epilepsy every year [2]. Epilepsy is a neurological disorder wherein there is an uncontrolled electrical discharge of neurons. Our whole brain is a biological neural network. The primary unit of the neurons system is the cell. Every neuron is made of two parts: axon and cell body dendrites. Neurons transmit signals throughout the body. Epilepsy can affect anyone at any stage of life. Epileptic patients experience a vast range of symptoms which largely depend on the portion and the area of the brain that is affected. Epileptic seizures are of potential harm since they are often responsible for physical, social consequences and psychological disorders, which may result in loss of consciousness, injury to the brain and, in certain cases, abrupt death [1].

Normally if seizure is found active in one section of the brain cell or tissue, then it may spread to remaining sections of the brain. If a clinical seizure were experienced by the patient, the neurologist would directly visualize and inspect whether the EEG signals are normal or abnormal [3, 4, 5, 6]. However, this process consumes too much time. Even an entire day may be insufficient to adequately visualize and inspect the patient reports. It may also require secondary neurology experts to help them in this area [7]. Although we are not replacing the neurologist expert, we can help them in reducing the time consumed for visualizing the report.

All activities occurring in our brain signals are detected by EEG. There are small metal discs or electrodes, which consists of wires that are to be placed on the scalp. The electrodes are mainly responsible for acquiring the electrical activity in form of signals from brain cells and hence mapping the pattern in the brain due to electrical activity. This is very efficient for diagnosis of several conditions ranging from minimal to severe harm like headaches, dizziness, epilepsy, sleeping disorders and deadly brain tumors. The very first EEG measurements were done by Hans Berger, who was a German psychiatrist, in the year 1929 [8]. EEG signals prove to be of great use in the detection of epileptic seizures since any rapid changes from the normal pattern could indicate the presence of a seizure. EEG signals get small-scale amplitudes of the order 20 μV [9]. The signals observed in the scalp are divided into four bands based on their frequencies namely: Delta in the range of 0.3–4 Hz; theta in the range of 4–8 Hz; alpha in the range of 8–13 Hz; and beta in the range of 13–30 Hz [8, 10]. An electrode is always placed in accordance with the 10–20 international system which is depicted in Figure 2.1. This system is used for electrode placement, where the respective electrode is placed at either (10 or 20) % of the total distance among the notion and the inion. In 10–20 placement, every electrode is marked with a letter and that followed by a number. Electrodes contain odd and even numbers. Odd numbers show that electrode is located on the left side of head. Even number shows that electrode is located on the right side of head. The letter indicates the area of the brain where the electrode is placed: F letter show that frontal lobe, T letter show that temporal lobe, P letter show that parietal and O letter show that occipital lobes, Letter Z denotes that the electrodes are positioned on the midline of the brain [11, 12].

Artificial Neural Networks (ANNs) were first developed several decades ago, by researchers attempting to develop the learning process of the human brain. ANN is typically composed of interconnected "units" which denote the modeled neurons [11, 12] in 2004, Nigam and Graupe [13, 14, 15, 16] presented a novel approach for the detection of epileptic seizures from the EEG recordings. It employs the Diagnosis of EEG signals of ANN in combination with a multistage nonlinear preprocessing filter. Kannathal et al. [12] Compared different entropy measures that are tested on EEG data and it has been proven that EEG data using ANFIS classifier have obtained an accuracy of 90%. Guo et al. [17] put forward a technique which uses Relative Wavelet Energy (RWE) for analysis of EEG signals which are then classified using ANNs. This method has achieved an accuracy of 95.20%. Homan et al. [18] in 2000 proposed an Epileptic Seizure Prediction system which depends on RNN. Guler et al. [60] proposed an EEG signal classification system that depends on Recurrent Neural Networks using Lyapunov exponents which has achieved an accuracy of up to 97.38%. Talathi [19] in 2017 presented an Epileptic

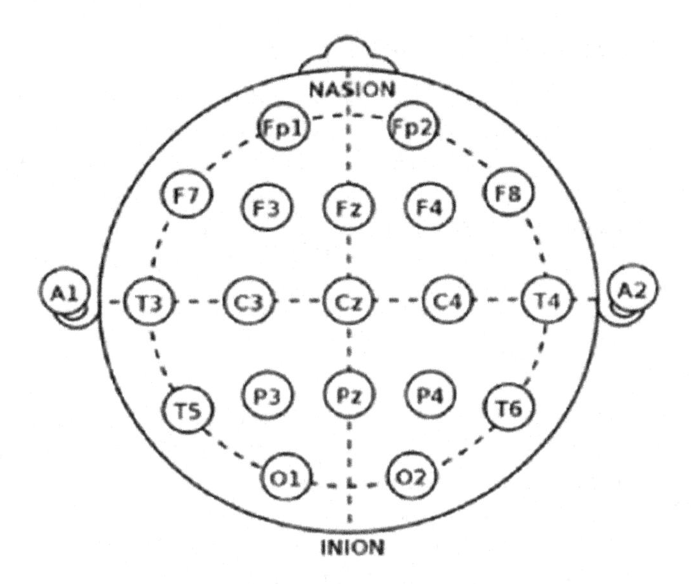

FIGURE 2.1 Standardized 10–20 electrode placement system.

Seizure Detection and classification established on Deep RNN which has obtained an accuracy of 99.6%. Nowadays, when millions of data comes into the clinical area for better accuracy, they use deep learning algorithms. Further Pereira et al. [20] have done automatic segmentation of brain tumors with the help of the convolutional neural network. Acharya et al. [21] in 2017 proposed an application that detection automated infraction using ECG signal that given 92.50% accuracy. Acharya et al. [22, 23] showed a deep Convolutional neural network in ECG signals for finding coronary artery disease that has acquired an accuracy of 94.95%.

ANN, which works on the idea of neural networks, is the backbone on which DL is based. For handling a gradient descent algorithm effectively, a back propagation algorithm is a very good approach which can be applied on any dataset. Although it has a very promising training accuracy, the testing accuracy seems detrimental. BPA faces the problem of local optima when its application is put to effect on random initialize node. In huge datasets, there is a problem of over-fitting as well. Henceforth, popular learning algorithms namely SVM, KNN, decision tree, and logistic regression are employed to achieve the global optima [3, 4, 24, 25].

The main contribution in the view of this paper, a novel deep CNN model is proposed for classifying EEG signals. In this model feature selection and extraction processes have been done automatically by convolutional and max-pooling layers. There is no requirement of any specific handcrafted feature extraction and selection technique, which also reduces the computational complexity of our model. In this model, first the Bonn university EEG database is normalized and then split into training and testing datasets. We have used 10-fold cross validations for dense layer and back propagation algorithm to classify the dataset into three classes normal, pre-ictal and epilepsy.

2.2 MATERIALS AND METHODOLOGY

In this area, we mainly describe the database and proposed methodology. A deep CNN model is used for classification of EEG signals. The dataset is classified into three distinct classes namely: normal, pre-ictal and seizure. The proposed work flow diagram for the detection of seizure patient is shown in the Figure 2.2. Then performance evaluation for different ratios like 90%, 80%, 70%, 60% of training and 10%, 20%, 30%, 40% testing respectively has been done. Also, 10-fold cross validation on 90-10 train test ratio was applied.

2.2.1 Dataset

The data taken by Andrzejak et al. [2] was used for research in this paper. The dataset has been obtained from 5 distinct patients that contain 3 different classes. There are normal (set-Z), Pre-ictal (set-N) and seizure (set-S). Each subset consists of 100 single-channel EEG fragments. Each fragment is of 23.6 s and has a sampling frequency of 173.6 Hz [10]. The complete EEG data was recorded using a 128-channel amplifier system, by employing an average common reference. The spectral bandwidth of the data ranges from 0.5 Hz to 85 Hz, which is similar to the acquisition system.

2.2.2 Normalization

In our study, the database has a mix of variables with large variance and small variance. Normalization is a radical transformation and is mainly done to get a normal distribution. For the normalization purpose, z-score normalization as a preprocessing step is extremely important for learning in the data preparation step. The main aim of normalization is to use a common scale by diverging the value of the numeric columns. The Z-score normalization is calculated according to equation 2.1, where μ is mean, σ is standard deviation and x is random variable.

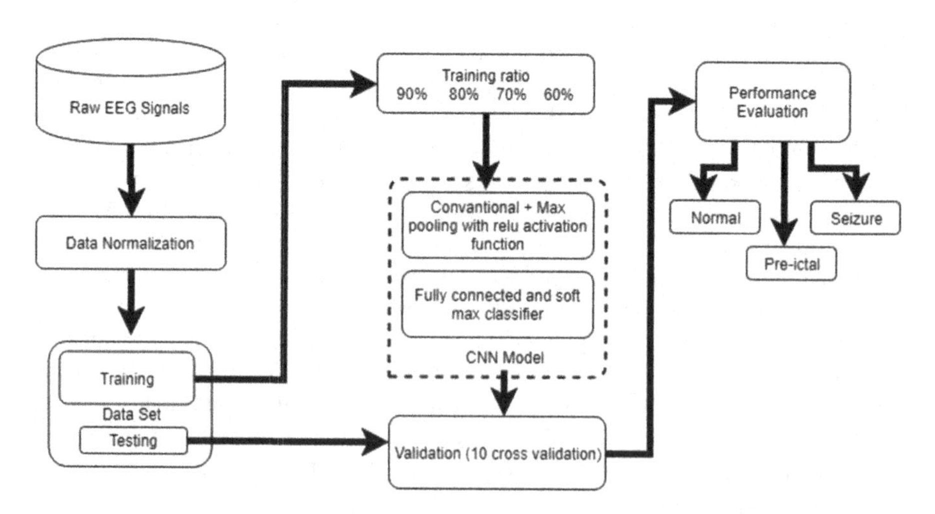

FIGURE 2.2 Flow chart of proposed model.

$$Z = \frac{(x - \mu)}{\sigma} \tag{2.1}$$

2.2.3 Convolution Neural Network (CNN)

Deep learning uses raw signal and extracts features automatically, directly from input data. The advantage that comes with DL is that these methods are more promising than any other classification method for big datasets. Here, the network keeps on learning to get the best weights. This is done by feedback sent from output periodically to update the weights until the best combination is found [26]. The basic ideology behind CNN is very much similar to LeNet-5. There are mainly 3 layers namely: convolutional layer, pooling layer and the fully connected layer [27, 28, 29].

***Convolutional layer*:** It is the primary or initial layer of the CNN model. Here, EEG signals along with the filters also called as kernels are taken as inputs and some special selected features are sent as output to the next layer. Each convolution is involved in getting a certain unique feature from the input values. [27, 30, 31].

Pooling Layer: Pooling operation is generally employed to reduce the dimensionality of the subsequent convolutional layer. For the same reason down sampling layer is used as an alias for this [24]. Average, max and sum pooling are the main distinct types of pooling. Generally, and most frequently, max pooling is used which has the role of finding the maximum elements for feature mapping process [32].

ReLU Function: In non-linear operation, ReLU is the abbreviation for Rectified Linear Unit. The function of ReLU is to map a negative value to zero and hence have all positive values so that the training can be fast and more effective [33]. It applies element-wise activation function [34, 35, 36], whose output is

$$f(y) = \begin{cases} 0, \& y < 0 \\ y, \& y \geq 0 \end{cases} \tag{2.2}$$

***Fully-Connected layer*:** The output to this layer is fed to this layer from the max-pooling layers. This layer is very much similar to a neural network [27]. The matrix in this layer is flattened and the formed vector is fed into a fully connected layer which resembles a neural network [37].

***SoftMax*:** It is the subsequent and the last output layer, which is used SoftMax activation function provides the end result in terms of classification [38, 39]. Mathematically it is represented as

$$\sigma(z)_i = \frac{e^{(z)_i}}{\sum_{j=1}^{k} e^{(z)_i}} \tag{2.3}$$

Proposed CNN Architecture Figure 2.3 below shows a summary of the architecture of the 12-layer proposed CNN model. There is a total of 4097 inputs and a combination of four convolutional layers, four max-pooling layers and three fully connected layers. For each convolutional layer, it is necessary to specify the filter

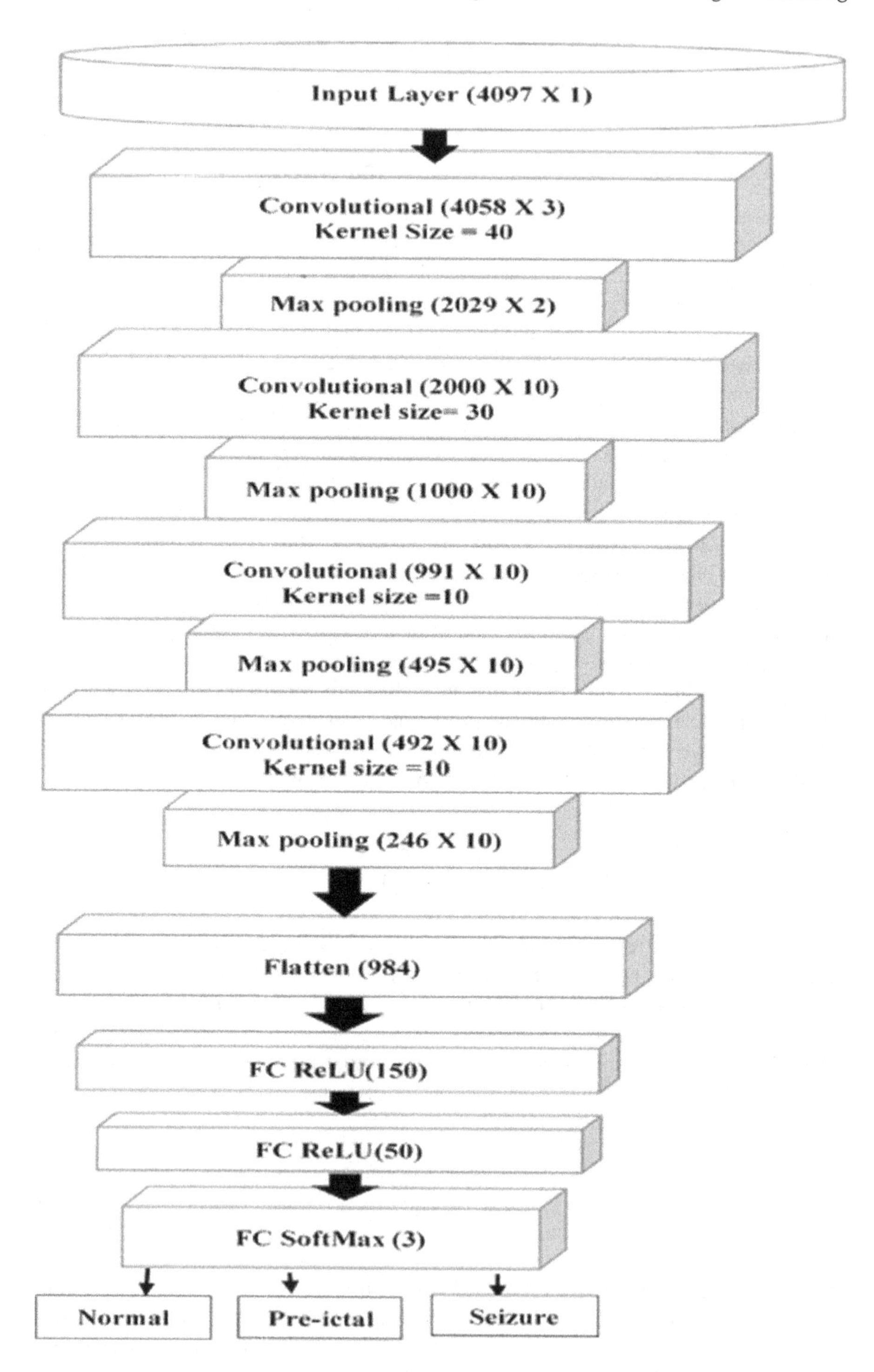

FIGURE 2.3 Architecture of proposed CNN model.

(kernel) size. The first convolutional layer is used at the kernel size 40 and returns the output data 4058, which is then passed to the maximum-pooling layer, which reduces the values to half of the convolutional layer and gives outputs 2029 values. The output of the max-pooling layer is passed to the second convolutional layer with filter size 30 and returns the output 2000 value, which is then passed to the max-pooling layer and produces an output 1000 data value. In addition, the third and fourth convolutional layer takes the input of 1000 and 495 data values with kernel size 10 and 4, with the latter max-pooling layer producing 991 and 492 data values, respectively. Flatten is employed for connecting the fully connected layer with ReLU activation function. Eventually, the ultimate three fully connected layers use SoftMax as the activation function.

2.3 RESULT AND DISCUSSIONS

2.3.1 Experiment 1: 10-Fold Cross Validation on 90:10 Ratio

In this proposed algorithm was implemented in python language with the help of keras libraries (https://keras.io/layers/convolutional). We take multiple simulations which were performed by varying the learning rate and the number of epochs to test our proposed method. We take all the ratios of training and testing. In our study, we employ 90% of data for training and the remaining 10% is used for validation procedures. Here, we have used a 10-fold cross-validation approach. Initially, the signals are randomly divided into 10 parts of equal ratio. Subsequently, 9 out of 10 signal fragments are used for training purpose. The remaining 1 portion of signal is used for validation of data. The explained strategy is used for different fragments and is repeated 10 times by using different training and testing data fragments. This works similar to the convolutional back propagation (BP) with a batch size of 34. Here, gradient of loss function is calculated with respect to the weight in the back-propagation procedure. This helps in giving backward feedback for error propagating in the network. At the time of training, weights are updated in a network. In this model, there exists a maximum of 50 epochs of training. 10% of the data is taken for testing. In 90% of data, it takes 70% of data for training and 30% of the remaining data for validations as shown in Figure 2.4.

Overall performance is evaluated on the basis of 3 main measurements namely: accuracy, specificity and sensitivity of the classification. All those measurements are described by using a confusion matrix. Where TP is for true positive, FP is for false positive, FN is for false negative and TN is for true negative [29].

$$\text{Accuracy} = \frac{(TP + TN)}{(TP + TN + FP + FN)} \tag{2.4}$$

$$\text{Sensitivity} = \frac{TP}{(TP + TN)} \tag{2.5}$$

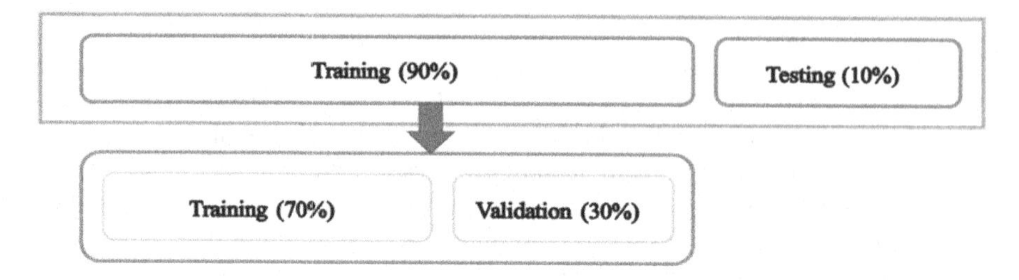

FIGURE 2.4 Data divided for training, validation, and testing ratios.

$$\text{Specificity} = \frac{TN}{(FPTN)} \tag{2.6}$$

$$\text{PPV} = \frac{TP}{(TP + FP)} \tag{2.7}$$

Table 2.1 presents the 90:10 ratio confusion matrix, for all ten-fold cross-validation. In this model we see that 95% are correctly classified as normal EEG signals and 5% are incorrectly classified. In pre-ictal class 97% of EEG signals are correctly classified and 3% are incorrectly classified. In seizure class 96% are correctly classified and 4% incorrectly classified.

Figure 2.5 depicts an accuracy graph for three class classifications, namely normal, pre-ictal and seizure class. Here the train test ratio is 90:10.

2.3.2 Experiment 2: Training and Testing Ratio Variation

Then we have performed training and testing with other ratios {like 80:20 ratio, 70:30 ratio, 60:40 ratio.} for this 12-layer deep CNN model. Then we present below tables.

Similarly, the Table 2.2 presents the 80:20 ratio confusion matrix. In this model we see that 99% has been correctly classified as normal EEG signal and 1% is incorrectly classified. While we consider the Pre-ictal class, 90% of EEG signals are

TABLE 2.1
Classification Results of Three Classes Using 10-Fold Cross Validation

	Predicted Normal	Pre-ictal	Seizure	Accuracy	PPV	Sensitivity	Specificity
Normal	95	3	2	97	95.95	95	98
Pre-ictal	2	97	1	97.33	95.09	97	97.5
Seizure	2	2	96	97.66	96.96	96	98.5

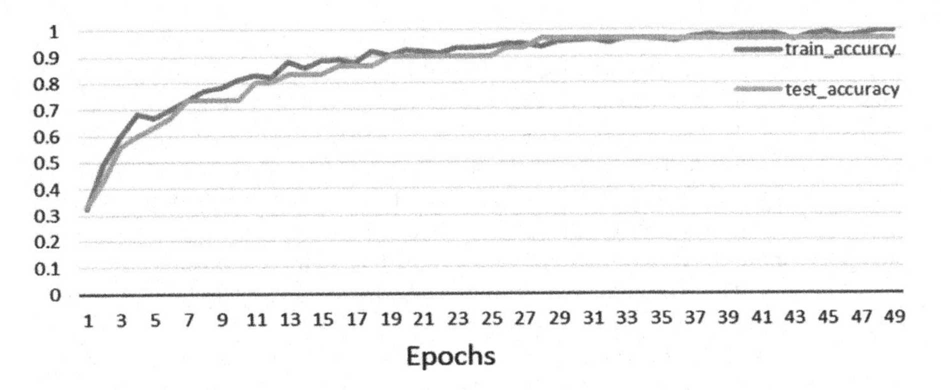

FIGURE 2.5 90:10 ratio training and testing accuracy graph for three classes.

TABLE 2.2
80:20 Ratio Confusion Matrix and Performance Summary

	Predicted Normal	Pre-ictal	Seizure	Accuracy	PPV	Sensitivity	Specificity
Normal	99	0	1	95.66	98.01	99	94
Pre-ictal	10	90	0	95.66	96.77	90	98.5
Seizure	2	3	95	98	98.95	95	99.5

correctly classified and 10% is incorrectly classified. And in case of the Seizure class, 95% of correct classified 5% incorrect classified.

The Table 2.3 presents the 70:30 ratio confusion matrix. In this model we see that 96% has been correctly classified as normal EEG signal and 4% is incorrectly classified. While we consider the Pre-ictal class, 98% of EEG signals are correct classified and 2% are incorrectly classified. And in case of the Seizure class 92% of correct classified 8% incorrect classified.

TABLE 2.3
70:30 Ration Confusion Matrix and Performance Summary

	Predicted Normal	Pre-ictal	Seizure	Accuracy	PPV	Sensitivity	Specificity
Normal	96	3	1	97.66	96.96	96	98.5
Pre-ictal	2	98	0	96	90.74	98	95.0
Seizure	1	7	92	97	98.92	92	99.5

Table 2.4 presents the 60:40 ratio confusion matrix. In this model we see that 78% have been correctly classified as Normal EEG signals and 22% are incorrectly classified. When we consider the Pre-ictal class, 98% of EEG signals are correctly classified and 2% are incorrectly classified. And in the case of the Seizure class 98% are correctly classified 2% incorrectly classified. We have acquired the best accuracy in the case of 90:10 train test ratio across 10-folds. The results were accuracy of 97.33%, sensitivity 96%, specificity 98% and precision 96%. The below table and graph show all types of training testing ratio done in this paper and performance evaluate them. The 10-fold cross validation performance results very well compared to other train-test ratios.

Table 2.5 shows the training accuracy and testing accuracy using different train test ratio with 50 epochs of the CNN model, and Figure 2.6 shows the graphical presentation of the testing accuracy.

Table 2.6 shows the computation and performance analysis of other research works. Nigam and Graupe [13] showed automated detection of epilepsy using neural network based from EEG signals. Firstly, non-linear prepossessing filter is applied that is a combination of the LAMSTAR neural network and ANN. Here, LAMSTAR is used for input preparation and ANN for training and system performance. In this paper, an accuracy of 97.20% was achieved. In a paper by Kannathal et al. [40, 41] worked in entropy estimated for detecting epileptic seizure in EEG signals. They have used ANFIS classifier for measuring test data. So the classification accuracy comes to

TABLE 2.4
60:40 Ratio Confusion Matrix and Performance Summary

	Predicted Normal	Pre-ictal	Seizure	Accuracy	PPV	Sensitivity	Specificity
Normal	78	22	0	91.33	98.74	78	99.00
Pre-ictal	2	98	0	91.33	80.32	98	88.00
Seizure	0	2	98	99.33	100	98	100

TABLE 2.5
All Ratio Training and Testing Performance

Ratio	Epochs	Training accuracy	Testing accuracy
90:10	50	99.83	97.33
80:20	50	99.12	95.00
70:30	50	98.75	92.00
60:40	50	98.33	90.50

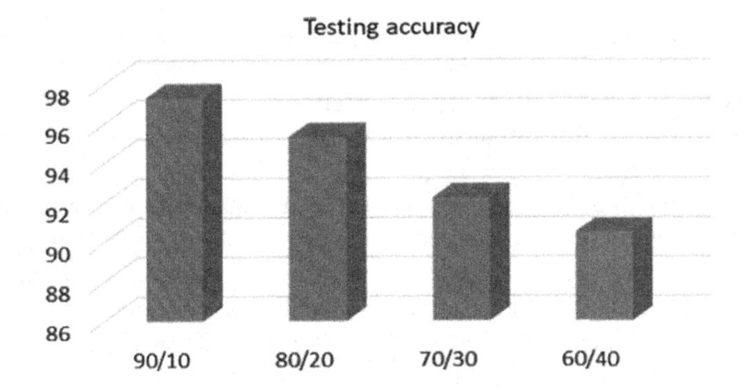

FIGURE 2.6 All ratio graph for testing accuracy.

TABLE 2.6
Synopsis of Erstwhile Research for Detection of Epileptic and Normal Classes

Author	Feature	Method	Accuracy (%)
Song and Liò [52]	Sample entropy	Extreme learning machine	95.67
Nigam and Graupe [13]	Nonlinear pre-processing filter	Diagnostic Neural Network	97.20
Kannathal et al. [40]	Entropy measures	ANFIS	92.20
Subasi [42]	DWT	Mixture expert model	94.50
Guo et al. [17]	DWT	MLPNN	95.20
Acharya et al. [53]	Entropy measures	Fuzzy logic	98.1
Chua et al. [54]; [55]	HOS and power spectral density	Gaussian classifier	93.11
Ubeyli et al. [56]; [57]	Wavelet transform	Mixture of expert model	93.17
Tawfik et al. [57]	Weighted Permutation Entropy	SVM	97.25
Ghosh-Dastidar et al. [59]	Nonlinear feature	Multi-spiking neural network	90.7 to 94.8
Acharya et al. [1]	10-fold cross validation strategy	13-layer CNN Model	88.7
Proposed model	10-fold cross validation strategy	12-layer CNN Model	ACC:97.33 SEN:96 SPE:98

90%. Subasi [42, 43, 44, 45, 46, 47, 48, 49, 50] in this paper uses DWT feature extraction in which the input taken EEG signals were decomposed into sub-bands. Then the sub-band was an input of a ME network for classification. An accuracy of 95% was obtained. Srinivasan et al. [51] in this study have used approximate entropy for feature extraction method. Approximate Entropy is the one that predicts the current amplitude values of a signal based on its previous values. The artificial neural network is used for classification of epilepsy class. Guo et al. [17] have done wavelet transforms that are derived from multi-wavelet transform as feature extraction and ANN for classification.

Song and Liò [52] proposed a novel method for automatic epileptic seizure detection. In this paper, they work on an optimized sample entropy algorithm for feature extraction. The extreme learning machine is used to identify the EEG recorded signal and determine whether it is normal or a seizure. Acharya et al. [53] proposed a method for automated detection of normal, pre-ictal and ictal conditions from EEG signal records. They take 4 entropy features that are sampEn, approximate entropy, phase entropy 1 and phase entropy 2. Then this feature extracted data was fed into 7 different types of classifiers: namely, SVM, Naive Bayes classifier, KNN, Gaussian mixture model, Decision tree, PNN, Fuzzy Sugeno entropy. Among the above mentioned seven classifiers Fuzzy classifier was able to differentiate into 3 classes with high efficiency.

2.4 CONCLUSION

In this paper, we have worked on the 12-layer CNN model for automated seizure detection employing the EEG signals. With reference to various popular methodologies, this study can perform better and hence effectively and accurately distinguish between the three classes: namely seizure, pre-ictal and normal EEG. The training and testing has been carried out on all the ratios, and we have observed that when the model is not obtaining a good percentage train data, it gives lower accuracy. The prime cause for lower accuracy is less percentage of train dataset. While learning, the model automatically performs feature extraction and selection process and hence acquires a greater number of data points for learning. Automated multiclass classification has been performed and has achieved an average accuracy of 97.33% with a specificity of 98% and a sensitivity of 96%. The proposed network has been applied and tested on the popular Bonn University EEG database and the performance has also been compared with various other baseline methods. The result clearly highlights the efficacy of the model in determining the efficiency, accuracy, and potential of the proposed study in detecting epileptic seizures. The added advantage with this study is that it automatically performs feature extraction and selection; hence there is no need for any specific methods. The advancement of the model's performance lies in testing it on more datasets.

REFERENCES

1. Acharya, U. Rajendra, Shu Lih Oh, Yuki Hagiwara, Jen Hong Tan, and Hojjat Adeli. 2018. Deep convolutional neural network for the automated detection and diagnosis of seizure using EEG signals. *Computers in Biology and Medicine* 100: 270–278.
2. Andrzejak, Ralph G., Klaus Lehnertz, Florian Mormann, Christoph Rieke, Peter David, and Christian E. Elger. 2001. Indications of nonlinear deterministic and finite-dimensional structures in time series of brain electrical activity: dependence on recording region and brain state. *Physical Review E* 64, no. 6: 061907.

3. Adeli, Hojjat, Ziqin Zhou, and Nahid Dadmehr. 2003. Analysis of EEG records in an epileptic patient using wavelet transform. *Journal of Neuroscience Methods* 123, no. 1: 69–87.
4. Marsan, C. Ajmone, and L. S. Zivin. 1970. Factors related to the occurrence of typical paroxysmal abnormalities in the EEG records of epileptic patients. *Epilepsia* 11, no. 4: 361–381.
5. Del Brutto, O. H., R. Santibanez, C. A. Noboa, R. Aguirre, E. Diaz, and T. A. Alarcon. 1992. Epilepsy due to neurocysticercosis: analysis of 203 patients. *Neurology* 42, no. 2: 389–389.
6. Salinsky, Martin, Roy Kanter, and Richard M. Dasheiff. 1987. Effectiveness of multiple EEGs in supporting the diagnosis of epilepsy: an operational curve. *Epilepsia* 28, no. 4: 331–334.
7. Mirowski, Piotr W., Yann LeCun, Deepak Madhavan, and Ruben Kuzniecky. 2008. Comparing SVM and convolutional networks for epileptic seizure prediction from intracranial EEG. In *2008 IEEE workshop on machine learning for signal processing*, pp. 244–249. IEEE.
8. Kallenberg, Michiel, Kersten Petersen, Mads Nielsen, Andrew Y. Ng, Pengfei Diao, Christian Igel, Celine M. Vachon et al. 2016. Unsupervised deep learning applied to breast density segmentation and mammographic risk scoring. *IEEE Transactions on Medical Imaging* 35, no. 5: 1322–1331.
9. Siddique, Nazmul, and Hojjat Adeli. 2013. Computational intelligence: Synergies of fuzzy logic, neural networks and evolutionary computing West Sussex, UK: Wiley.
10. Selvan, S., and R. Srinivasan. 1999. Removal of ocular artifacts from EEG using an efficient neural network based adaptive filtering technique. *IEEE Signal Processing Letters* 6, no. 12: 330–332.
11. Agarwal, Rajeev, Jean Gotman, Danny Flanagan, and Bernard Rosenblatt. 1998. Automatic EEG analysis during long-term monitoring in the ICU. *Electroencephalography and Clinical Neurophysiology* 107, no. 1: 44–58.
12. Kannathal, N., Min Lim Choo, U. Rajendra Acharya, and P. K. Sadasivan. 2005. Entropies for detection of epilepsy in EEG. *Computer Methods and Programs in Biomedicine* 80, no. 3: 187–194.
13. Nigam, Vivek Prakash, and Daniel Graupe. 2004. A neural-network-based detection of epilepsy. *Neurological Research* 26, no. 1: 55–60.
14. Tzallas, Alexandros T., Markos G. Tsipouras, and Dimitrios I. Fotiadis. 2009. Epileptic seizure detection in EEGs using time–frequency analysis. *IEEE Transactions on Information Technology in Biomedicine* 13, no. 5: 703–710.
15. Omerhodzic, Ibrahim, Samir Avdakovic, Amir Nuhanovic, and Kemal Dizdarevic. 2013. Energy distribution of EEG signals: EEG signal wavelet-neural network classifier. *arXiv preprint arXiv:1307.7897.*
16. Puthankattil, Subha D., and Paul K. Joseph. 2012. Classification of EEG signals in normal and depression conditions by ANN using RWE and signal entropy. *Journal of Mechanics in Medicine and Biology* 12, no. 04: 1240019.
17. Guo, Ling, Daniel Rivero, Jose A. Seoane, and Alejandro Pazos. 2009. Classification of EEG signals using relative wavelet energy and artificial neural networks. In *Proceedings of the first ACM/SIGEVO Summit on Genetic and Evolutionary Computation*, pp. 177–184. ACM.
18. Petrosian, Arthur, Danil Prokhorov, Richard Homan, Richard Dasheiff, and Donald Wunsch II. 2000. Recurrent neural network based prediction of epileptic seizures in intra-and extracranial EEG. *Neurocomputing* 30, no. 1–4: 201–218.
19. Talathi, Sachin S. 2017. Deep Recurrent Neural Networks for seizure detection and early seizure detection systems. *arXiv preprint arXiv:1706.03283.*

20. Havaei, Mohammad, Axel Davy, David Warde-Farley, Antoine Biard, Aaron Courville, Yoshua Bengio, Chris Pal, Pierre-Marc Jodoin, and Hugo Larochelle. 2017. Brain tumor segmentation with deep neural networks. *Medical Image Analysis* 35: 18–31.
21. Acharya, U. Rajendra, Hamido Fujita, Oh Shu Lih, Yuki Hagiwara, Jen Hong Tan, and Muhammad Adam. 2017. Automated detection of arrhythmias using different intervals of tachycardia ECG segments with convolutional neural network. *Information Sciences* 405: 81–90.
22. Acharya, U. Rajendra, Hamido Fujita, Oh Shu Lih, Muhammad Adam, Jen Hong Tan, and Chua Kuang Chua. 2017. Automated detection of coronary artery disease using different durations of ECG segments with convolutional neural network. *Knowledge-Based Systems* 132: 62–71.
23. Cecotti, Hubert, and Axel Graser. 2010. Convolutional neural networks for P300 detection with application to brain-computer interfaces. *IEEE Transactions on Pattern Analysis and Machine Intelligence* 33, no. 3: 433–445.
24. Pereira, Sérgio, Adriano Pinto, Victor Alves, and Carlos A. Silva. 2016. Brain tumor segmentation using convolutional neural networks in MRI images. *IEEE Transactions on Medical Imaging* 35, no. 5: 1240–1251.
25. Pandey, Saroj Kumar, and Rekh Ram Janghel. 2019. Recent deep learning techniques, challenges and its applications for medical healthcare system: a review. *Neural Processing Letters* 50: 1–29.
26. Bar, Yaniv, Idit Diamant, Lior Wolf, and Hayit Greenspan. 2015. Deep learning with non-medical training used for chest pathology identification. In *Medical Imaging 2015: Computer-Aided Diagnosis*, vol. 9414, p. 94140V. International Society for Optics and Photonics.
27. Shin, Hoo-Chang, Holger R. Roth, Mingchen Gao, Le Lu, Ziyue Xu, Isabella Nogues, Jianhua Yao, Daniel Mollura, and Ronald M. Summers. 2016. Deep convolutional neural networks for computer-aided detection: CNN architectures, dataset characteristics and transfer learning. *IEEE Transactions on Medical Imaging* 35, no. 5: 1285–1298.
28. Zhang, Kai, Wangmeng Zuo, Yunjin Chen, Deyu Meng, and Lei Zhang. 2017. Beyond a gaussian denoiser: residual learning of deep cnn for image denoising. *IEEE Transactions on Image Processing* 26, no. 7: 3142–3155.
29. Pandey, Saroj Kumar, and Rekh Ram Janghel. 2019. ECG Arrhythmia Classification Using Artificial Neural Networks. In *Proceedings of 2nd International Conference on Communication, Computing and Networking*, pp. 645–652. Springer, Singapore.
30. Milletari, Fausto, Seyed-Ahmad Ahmadi, Christine Kroll, Annika Plate, Verena Rozanski, Juliana Maiostre, Johannes Levin et al. 2017. Hough-CNN: deep learning for segmentation of deep brain regions in MRI and ultrasound. *Computer Vision and Image Understanding* 164: 92–102.
31. Zhou, Bolei, Agata Lapedriza, Jianxiong Xiao, Antonio Torralba, and Aude Oliva. 2014. Learning deep features for scene recognition using places database. In *Advances in neural information processing systems*, pp. 487–495.
32. Wu, Zuxuan, Xi Wang, Yu-Gang Jiang, Hao Ye, and Xiangyang Xue. 2015. Modeling spatial-temporal clues in a hybrid deep learning framework for video classification. In *Proceedings of the 23rd ACM international conference on Multimedia*, pp. 461–470. ACM.
33. Sharif Razavian, Ali, Hossein Azizpour, Josephine Sullivan, and Stefan Carlsson. 2014. CNN features off-the-shelf: an astounding baseline for recognition. In *Proceedings of the IEEE conference on computer vision and pattern recognition workshops*, pp. 806–813.

34. Goodfellow, Ian, Yoshua Bengio, and Aaron Courville. 2016. *Deep learning.* Cambridge: MIT Press.
35. Litjens, Geert, Thijs Kooi, Babak Ehteshami Bejnordi, Arnaud Arindra Adiyoso Setio, Francesco Ciompi, Mohsen Ghafoorian, Jeroen Awm Van Der Laak, Bram Van Ginneken, and Clara I. Sánchez. 2017. A survey on deep learning in medical image analysis. *Medical Image Analysis* 42: 60–88.
36. Feng, Minwei, Bing Xiang, Michael R. Glass, Lidan Wang, and Bowen Zhou. 2015. Applying deep learning to answer selection: a study and an open task. In *2015 IEEE Workshop on Automatic Speech Recognition and Understanding (ASRU)*, pp. 813–820. IEEE.
37. Bashivan, Pouya, Irina Rish, Mohammed Yeasin, and Noel Codella. 2015. Learning representations from EEG with deep recurrent-convolutional neural networks. *arXiv preprint arXiv:1511.06448.*
38. He, Kaiming, Xiangyu Zhang, Shaoqing Ren, and Jian Sun. 2015. Delving deep into rectifiers: surpassing human-level performance on imagenet classification. In *Proceedings of the IEEE international conference on computer vision*, pp. 1026–1034.
39. Hung, Shih-Lin, and Hojjat Adeli. 1993. Parallel backpropagation learning algorithms on Cray Y-MP8/864 supercomputer. *Neurocomputing* 5, no. 6: 287–302.
40. Kannathal, N., Min Lim Choo, U. Rajendra Acharya, and P. K. Sadasivan. 2005. Entropies for detection of epilepsy in EEG. *Computer Methods and Programs in Biomedicine* 80, no. 3: 187–194.
41. Sadati, Nasser, Hamid Reza Mohseni, and Arash Maghsoudi. 2006. Epileptic seizure detection using neural fuzzy networks. In *2006 IEEE international conference on fuzzy systems*, pp. 596–600. IEEE.
42. Subasi, Abdulhamit. 2007. EEG signal classification using wavelet feature extraction and a mixture of expert model. *Expert Systems with Applications* 32, no. 4: 1084–1093.
43. Cho, Kyunghyun, Bart Van Merriënboer, Dzmitry Bahdanau, and Yoshua Bengio. 2014. On the properties of neural machine translation: encoder-decoder approaches. *arXiv preprint arXiv:1409.1259.*
44. Shickel, Benjamin, Patrick James Tighe, Azra Bihorac, and Parisa Rashidi. 2017. Deep EHR: a survey of recent advances in deep learning techniques for electronic health record (EHR) analysis. *IEEE Journal of Biomedical and Health Informatics* 22, no. 5: 1589–1604.
45. Acharya, U. Rajendra, Filippo Molinari, S. Vinitha Sree, Subhagata Chattopadhyay, Kwan-Hoong Ng, and Jasjit S. Suri. 2012. Automated diagnosis of epileptic EEG using entropies. *Biomedical Signal Processing and Control* 7, no. 4: 401–408.
46. Sharma, Manish, Ram Bilas Pachori, and U. Rajendra Acharya. 2017. A new approach to characterize epileptic seizures using analytic time-frequency flexible wavelet transform and fractal dimension. *Pattern Recognition Letters* 94: 172–179.
47. Cortes, Corinna, and Vladimir Vapnik. 1995. Support-vector networks. *Machine Learning* 20, no. 3: 273–297.
48. Srinivasan, Vairavan, Chikkannan Eswaran, and Natarajan Sriraam. 2007. Approximate entropy-based epileptic EEG detection using artificial neural networks. *IEEE Transactions on Information Technology in Biomedicine* 11, no. 3: 288–295.
49. Nigam, Vivek Prakash, and Daniel Graupe. 2004. A neural-network-based detection of epilepsy. *Neurological Research* 26, no. 1: 55–60.
50. Sadati, Nasser, Hamid Reza Mohseni, and Arash Maghsoudi. 2006. Epileptic seizure detection using neural fuzzy networks. In *2006 IEEE international conference on fuzzy systems*, pp. 596–600. IEEE.
51. Srinivasan, Vairavan, Chikkannan Eswaran, and Natarajan Sriraam. 2007. Approximate entropy-based epileptic EEG detection using artificial neural networks. *IEEE Transactions on Information Technology in Biomedicine* 11, no. 3: 288–295.

52. Song, Yuedong, and Pietro Liò. 2010. A new approach for epileptic seizure detection: sample entropy-based feature extraction and extreme learning machine. Journal of Biomedical Science and Engineering 3, no. 06: 556.
53. Acharya, U. Rajendra, Filippo Molinari, S. Vinitha Sree, Subhagata Chattopadhyay, Kwan-Hoong Ng, and Jasjit S. Suri. 2012. Automated diagnosis of epileptic EEG using entropies. *Biomedical Signal Processing and Control* 7, no. 4: 401–408.
54. Chua, Kuang Chua, Vinod Chandran, U. Rajendra Acharya, and Choo Min Lim. 2011. Application of higher order spectra to identify epileptic EEG. *Journal of Medical Systems* 35, no. 6: 1563–1571.
55. Rohit Raja, Sandeep Kumar, and Md Rashid. Color object detection based image retrieval using ROI segmentation with multi-feature method. Wireless Personal Communication Springer Journal, https://doi.org/10.1 007/s11277-019-07021-6.
56. Rohit Raja, Tilendra Shishir Sinha, Raj Kumar Patra, and Shrikant Tiwari. 2018. Physiological trait based biometrical authentication of human-face using LGXP and ANN techniques. International Journal of Information and Computer Security 10, no. 2/3: 303–320.
57. Tawfik, Noha S., Sherin M. Youssef, and Mohamed Kholief. 2016. A hybrid automated detection of epileptic seizures in EEG records. *Computers & Electrical Engineering* 53: 177–190.
58. Güler, Nihal Fatma, Elif Derya Übeyli, and Inan Güler. 2005. Recurrent neural networks employing Lyapunov exponents for EEG signals classification. *Expert Systems with Applications* 29, no. 3: 506–514.
59. Ghosh-Dastidar, Samanwoy, and Hojjat Adeli. 2009. A new supervised learning algorithm for multiple spiking neural networks with application in epilepsy and seizure detection. *Neural Networks* 22, no. 10: 1419–1431.

3 Medical Image De-Noising Using Combined Bayes Shrink and Total Variation Techniques

Devanand Bhonsle, G. R. Sinha, and Vivek Kumar Chandra

CONTENTS

3.1 INTRODUCTION

In the present era images have many applications; for example, law enforcement, biometrics, remote sensing, medical science and so on (Gonzalez and Woods, 2009).

Medical imaging deals with various types of images which are used in medical fields. Examples of medical images (Gravel et al., 2004) are CT images (Attivissimo et al., 2010; Petrongolo and Zhu, 2015), X-ray images, MRI, US images and so on which are used in the diagnostic process by radiologists for the detection and analysis of abnormalities in the human body (Patel and Sinha, 2014). The image data may be degraded due to several factors and various natural phenomena. To capture the images, various instruments are to be used. These instruments are not always perfect and they may reduce the quality of captured images. Some problems occur during the acquisition process which may further degrade the quality of images. Medical imaging systems are more accurate and they provide good quality of medical images but they may also be corrupted due to natural phenomena (Raj and Venkateswarlu, 2011; Trinh et al., 2014). Medical images are affected by various noise signals; namely Gaussian noise (Flower, 2005), Rician, speckle and so on and quality of images may be corrupted. As a consequence, false interpretations can be made by the radiologists. Hence, suppression of noise signals is essential before analyzing these images. De-noising is a preprocessing task in the field of image processing. De-noising is done not only to suppress noise signals, but also to preserve the useful information of the images such as edges, fine structures, texture details and so on (Choubey et al., 2011). Many methods have been implemented for image de-noising but no method provides satisfactory results for different types of noise problems. Hence a framework has been developed which suppresses noise signals and preserves image information (Sheikh and Bovik, 2006).

Image is a 2D function $x(i, j)$; where i and j are spatial coordinates. For any pixel coordinate (i, j); amplitude of x is called gray value of the image which is sometimes referred as the amplitude of x (Gonzalez and Woods, 2009). If the values of pixel coordinates and the amplitudes of x both are discrete and finite quantities then the image is called a digital image. Various medical images are Positron Emission Tomography (PET) images, CT images (Kumar and Diwakar, 2018), X-ray images, MRI, US images and so on. In this chapter a novel framework is proposed to de-noise CT images and suppresses Gaussian noise effectively.

CT images are widely used in the medical field to detect various types of diseases such as lung cancer and so on. The introduction of noise is a universal problem in CT imaging (Iborra et al., 2015). CT imaging systems require doses of radiation. Higher radiation doses increase the risk of cancer. Therefore, it must be reduced to a certain extent. However, low doses may cause poor quality of images (Hashemi et al., 2015) as it may produce noisy images which may affect the diagnosis process and may lead to false interpretations by the radiologists (Kumar and Diwakar, 2018).

Let us consider that the original image x(i, j) is corrupted by noise signal n(i, j); as a result, noise image y(i, j) is obtained. Since noise is additive hence

$$y(i, j) = x(i, j) + n(i, j) \tag{3.1}$$

Gaussian noise is also known as white noise because it is evenly distributed over the signal. If this noise is introduced in any image, then the noisy image contains noisy pixels. The noise pixel is the sum of actual pixel value and the Gaussian noise values. Noise is randomly distributed over the image. Figure 3.3 illustrates the

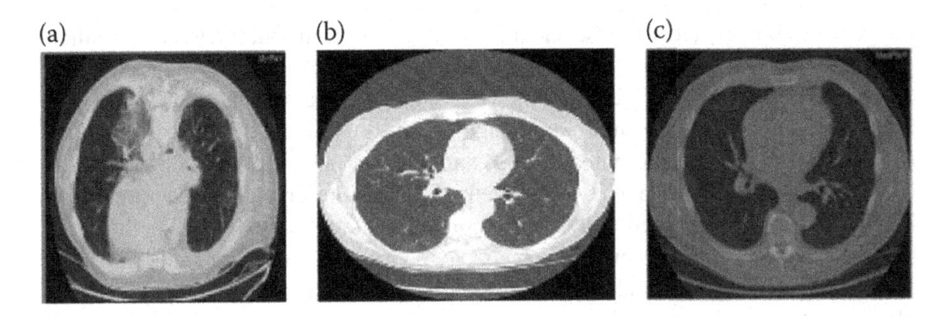

FIGURE 3.1 CT images.

Probability Distribution Function (PDF) of the additive Gaussian noise which is bell shaped. The PDF of Gaussian noise is given by:

$$f(g) = \frac{1}{\sqrt{2\pi\sigma^2}} e^{-(g-m)^2/2\sigma^2} \quad (3.2)$$

3.2 LITERATURE REVIEW

This part provides a brief overview of previous research done on image de-noising. Much research has been done in this field and many techniques have been implemented. The main goal of all these techniques is to improve the image quality and to retain information such as edges, fine structures, texture details and so on. AWGN noise affects almost all the frequency bands. (Gravel et al., 2004) presented a technique to model noises in images used in the medical field. It is known that CT images may be severely affected by AWGN; speckle is the inherent property of US images, while MRI images are affect by Rician noise. Below is the description of different approaches proposed in various research papers.

(Aggarwal and Majumdar, 2015) addressed the problem to reduce the effect of mixed noise from hyper-spectral images. Mixed noise is the mixture of Gaussian and impluse noise signals which is introduced during the data acquisition process. In this method; the split-Bregman approach is used to solve the resulting optimization problem [1]. (Aggarwal et al., 2016) introduced a SSTV technique to reduce mixed noise from the hyperspectral images. In this method, the de-noising problem is considered as an optimization problem and the solution is obtained using the split-Bregman approach [2]. (Ahmad et al., 2012) proposed hybrid estimated threshold to remove three types of noise signals; namely speckle, Gaussians, and salt and pepper from US images. It combines shrinkage technique with translation invariant and block function in the wavelet domain. It performs well enough to remove salt and pepper noise. It keeps the brightness and background, as well as gray level tonalities in medical images [3]. (Ali and Sukanesh, 2011) presented a curvelet-based technique to de-noise medical images such as MRI and CT images. It is applied to remove white, poisson and random noise. Curvelet transform exhibits better performance than wavelet-based transform in terms of visual quality.

Images are sharper and have better quality edges. Overall, curvelet-based method provides better de-noising [4]. (Attivissimo et al., 2010) proposed a method for de-noising CT images by combining Gaussian and Prewitt operators with AD technique. This technique improves image quality of low dose CT images [5, 6]. (Borsdorf et al., 2008) presented a noise suppression method which de-noises CT images efficiently. It is wavelet-based method, which preserves the structure of CT images. It can be combined with other reconstruction methods. In this method it is assumed that any data either signal or image can be decomposing into two parts, specifically information and noise signals. It is a robust method with low complexity and it can adapt itself according to the noise signal present in the image [7]. (Cannistraci et al., 2009) proposed Median Modified Wiener Filter (MMWF), which is an adaptive non-linear filter in spatial domain. It has the ability to remove spikes completely and Gaussian noise partially; hence, it is known as a global de-noising filter. The advantages of this method are that it preserves the useful information and does not suffer from erosion. It can be consider ed the best filter if the goal is to minimize spot edge aberration while removing Gaussian noise and spikes from the images [8]; [9]. (Cong-Hua et al., 2014) proposed a method to de-noise medical images which uses a Gaussian mixture model. This method preserves the edge information [10]; [11]. (Eng and Ma, 2001) implemented Median Filter (MF) based on switching, which also includes the concepts of fuzzy set. It is known as noise adaptive soft switching MF. It removes impulse noise efficiently and preserves signal details [12, 13]. (Goldstein and Osher, 2009) demonstrated that Bregman iteration has a capability to solve a variety of constrained optimization issues in different fields. Split-Bregman approach is used to suppress the noise present in images [14, 15]. (Gravel et al., 2004) explained the statistical properties of noise which may be present in medical images. The noise signals may originate from many factors. They are generally introduced during the acquisition of the images and not generated due to tissue textures. Generally, noise signals are considered additive noise having Gaussian distribution, but noise variance can be modeled using non-linear function which may depend on image intensity. This model helps us to find the relationship between noise variance and image intensity [16, 17, 18, 19, 20, 21]. (Huang et al., 2009) proposed an image restoration technique for images affected by impulse noise or mixed noise. An image can be corrupted by more than one noise. For example, the noise may be the mixture of Gaussian and impulsive noise or Gaussian and speckle noise. For the proposed technique, mixed noise is considered the combination of Gaussian and salt and pepper noise. For this mixed noise problem, modified Total Variation (TV) technique is used. MF is used to detect those pixels that are affected by noise signal. Noisy pixel can be replaced by a suitable pixel after detection [22]. (Huo et al., 2016) addressed the ringing artifacts problem in CT images which is introduced due to the inconsistent response of detector pixels. To remove this effect, a unidirectional relative variation model is used [23, 24]. (Ioannidou and Karathanassi, 2007) investigated performance of shift invariant discrete wavelet transform (DWT) and DTCWT in Quick-bird image fusion technique. It is applied on high resolution muiti-spectral Quick-bird images. To evaluate the effectiveness of this method, performances for various existing techniques are compared with it [25].

Conventional DWT suffers from two drawbacks which have been resolved by introducing DTCWT (Kingsbury, 1998) because DTCWT is nearly shift-invariant and it exhibits good directional property for two as well as higher dimensions [26, 27]. (Kingsbury, 2000) presented another form of the DTCWT which has improved orthogonality as well as symmetry properties. It consists of an even length filer which has asymmetric coefficients. The design makes it suitable for multi-dimensional signals [28]. (Kingsbury, 2001) described a form of DWT based on a dual tree of wavelet filters. It provides real and imaginary parts from complex coefficients. DTCWT overcomes the shift variance and poor directional property of DWT. It is suitable for two dimensional and can be further extended for multi-dimensional signals [29] (Kingsbury, 1998) presented an implementation of the DWT for image de-noising and image enhancement which is known as DTCWT. It introduces less redundancy. For m dimensional signals redundancy is only 2^m: 1. It offers high computational efficiency and perfect reconstruction. It provides good platform for de-noising and de-blurring for two and multi-dimensional signals [30, 31, 32, 33, 34, 35]. (Miller and Kingsbury, 2008) proposed AWGN removal technique, which uses the statistical modeling of coefficients of a redundant, oriented and complex multi-scale transform. The proposed algorithm uses two different forms of modeling which are derived from Gaussian scale mixture modeling of neighborhoods of coefficients at adjacent locations and scales. It reduces ringing artifacts, enhances sharpness and avoids degradation in other areas [36, 37, 38, 39, 40]. (Sapthagirivasan and Mahadevan, 2010) presented a DTCWT based automatic method for de-noising and segmentation of lung lobes using high resolution CT images [41]. (Sendur and Selesnick, 2002) presented an adaptive technique for de-noising using bivariate thresholding which can be applied using both the orthogonal and DTCWT. The performance is to be enhanced using simple models by estimating the model parameters in a local neighborhood [42, 43, 44, 45, 46, 47, 48, 49]

After a review of various literatures, it may be concluded that noise is a general problem in images because it degrades the quality by suppressing important features. Hence, it is important to remove the noise signals or reduce their effect in the images. The main goal of de-noising is not only the suppression of noise, but also the preservation of as much important image information as possible. Wavelet based de-noising methods provide better performance than many other techniques. The most popular wavelet transform is DTCWT, which provides many advantages which are required for image processing. De-noising using WT requires a thresholding technique in which noisy coefficients are either removed or replaced by the calculated value. Many thresholding techniques have been proposed, specifically neigh shrink, sure shrink, Vishu shrink, Bayes shrink and so on. Adaptive thresholding techniques provide better results than the non-adaptive thresholding techniques. TV techniques are non-wavelet methods, which provide good de-noising results for mixed noise problems.

3.3 THEORETICAL ANALYSIS

The proposed framework consists of MF-, MMWF-, DTCWT-based bivariate thresholding technique and the TV method. Adaptive thresholding and the TV method are applied in parallel, which provide two de-noised images that are fused together using DTCWT based fusion technique (Li et al., 2012). This procedure is called "Shrinkage Combined Enhanced Total Variation" (SCETV) method. In this chapter we provide a description of various filters which have been used to design our framework.

3.3.1 Median Modified Wiener Filter

Median Modified Wiener Filter (MMWF) may be considered the best filter for image de-noising because it can remove various types of noise signals (Cannistraci et al., 2009). It is the best choice among the filters available as it minimizes the spot edge aberrations while suppressing salt and pepper noise and/or white Gaussian noise. It is an example of a nonlinear adaptive filter which adapted qualities of both Median Filter (MF) and Wiener Filter (WF). It removes salt and pepper noise while preserving unaltered spot edges. For an image with the size $M \times N$ of the local neighborhood area η contained in the kernel, the estimate of local (considered in kernel) mean μ and variance σ^2 around each pixel in the image is given by equation (3.1) and equation (3.2) respectively.

$$\mu = \sum_{m,n \in \eta} a(m, n) \tag{3.1}$$

$$\sigma^2 = \frac{1}{M \times N} \sum_{m,n \in \eta} a^2(m, n) - \mu^2 \tag{3.2}$$

In WF implementation; the new pixel values $b_{WF}(m, n)$ may be estimated as:

$$b_{WF}(m, n) = \mu + \frac{\sigma^2 - v^2}{\sigma^2} \{a(m, n) - \mu\} \tag{3.3}$$

The modification in WF concerns the local kernel mean value around each pixelv μ. In MMWF μ is replaced with μ' which is estimation of local kernel median around each pixel. The new pixel value $b_{MMWF}(m,n)$ is given as:

$$b_{MMWF}(m, n) = \mu' + \frac{\sigma^2 - v^2}{\sigma^2} \{a(m, n) - \mu'\} \tag{3.4}$$

3.3.2 Wavelet Transform

DWT is an effective tool in many application areas. The most common area is image processing. Its performance is better than many other non-wavelet techniques. However, its performance is hampered due to two problems; namely, shift variance and poor directional property. To avoid these major drawbacks, complex wavelet filters can be used which improve shift invariance property and directional property. However, implementation of these filters is difficult and hence they cannot be used widely.

3.3.3 Dual Tree Complex Wavelet Transform

To overcome the aforementioned problem of DWT, (Kingsbury, 1998) proposed Dual Tree Complex Wavelet Transform (DTCWT) which consists of two parallel DWT filter banks. This structure of DTCWT generates the wavelet coefficients differently. DTCWT is the modification of DWT by which Complex coefficients are generated using dual tree wavelet filters which provide their real and imaginary parts. DTCWT can decompose any image into complex sub-images in different levels. It contains 6 oriented sub-images, resulting from evenly spaced directional filtering and sub-sampling. These coefficients are used for the computation of amplitude and phase information.

3.3.4 Sure Shrink

SURE Shrink minimizes MSE and suppresses noise signals by thresholding the empirical wavelet coefficients. SURE, shrink is given as:

$$t* = \min(t, \sigma\sqrt{2\log n}) \tag{3.5}$$

where t is the value which minimizes SURE, σ is the noise variance.

An estimate of the noise level σ is given as:

$$\hat{\sigma} = \frac{median(\{|g_{j-1,k}|: k = 0, 1 \ldots\ldots .2^{j-1} - 1\})}{0.6745} \tag{3.6}$$

3.3.5 Bayes Shrink

Bayes Shrink is proposed by Chang, Yu and Vetterli [50]. It minimizes Baysian risk hence it is named as Bayes shrink. The Bayes threshold t_B is given as

$$t_B = \frac{\sigma^2}{\sigma_s} \tag{3.7}$$

where σ^2 is called noise variance and σ_s called signal variance without noise.

3.3.6 Neigh Shrink

In Neigh Shrink thresholding, we have to consider neighborhood window $B_{j,k}$ around every coefficient $d_{j,k}$. The minimum window size is 3 × 3. Other sizes are 5 × 5, 7 × 7, 9 × 9 etc. Let

$$S_{j,k}^2 = \Sigma_{(i,l)\in B_{j,k}} d_{i,l}^2 \tag{3.8}$$

The shrinkage factor can be defined as:

$$\beta_{j,k} = (1 - \lambda^2 / S_{j,k}^2)_+ \tag{3.9}$$

where $\lambda = \sqrt{2\sigma^2 \log N^2}$.

Positive (+) indicates that we have to keep the positive value and set it to zero if negative value is obtained.

3.3.7 DTCWT Based De-Noising Using Adaptive Thresholding

As already mentioned, DTCWT performs better than conventional DWT; hence to get better performance DWT is replaced by DTCWT. Figure 3.2 shows a block diagram of DTCWT-based image de-noising technique using thresholding function.

There are three steps only:

i. Calculate DTCWT of noisy image.
ii. Modify noisy wavelet coefficients using bivariate thresholding.
iii. Compute IDTCWT to get de-noised image.

3.4 TOTAL VARIATION TECHNIQUE

(Aggarwal and Majumdar, 2016) proposed a technique to suppress mixed noise from hyperspectral images using SSTV method which exploits the spatial as well as spectral correlation present in the neighboring bands of the images. Let us consider an image in which mixed noise has been introduced. Then the noisy image can be expressed as:

$$y = x + n_{sp} + g \tag{3.10}$$

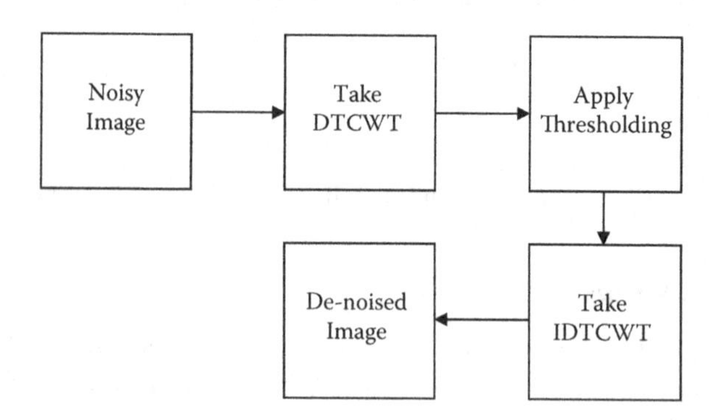

FIGURE 3.2 Additive noise removal technique using DTCWT based bivariate thresholding.

where, x, y n_{sp} and g represent original image, noisy image, salt and pepper and Gaussian noise respectively.

Generally, pixels are spatially correlated to their neighboring pixels values. This characteristic can be exploited to represent an image as piecewise smooth function and an image can be modeled using TV regularization. Let us consider a grayscale image is x. The SSTV model exploits both spatial and spectral correlation and it may be given as:

$$SSTV(x) = \|d_h x d\|_1 + \|d_v x d\|_1 \quad (3.11)$$

where d_h is horizontal and d_v is vertical 2D finite differencing operator.

d is a 1D finite differencing operator.

In SSTV model, de-noising problem is given as:

$$\min_{x,\, n_{sp}} \|y - x - n_{sp}\|_F^2 + \lambda\|n_{sp}\|_1 + \mu SSTV(x) \quad (3.12)$$

where, λ and μ are regularization parameters.

From equation (3.29)

$$g = y - x - n_{sp} \quad (3.13)$$

From equation (3.32) it is clear that the effect of Gaussian noise can be minimized by minimizing the Fresenius norm of $y - x - n_{sp}$

De-noising algorithm:

From equation (3.30) and equation (3.31), the de-noising problem can be given as:

$$\min_{x,\, n_{sp}} \|y - x - n_{sp}\|_F^2 + \lambda\|n_{sp}\|_1 + \mu\|d_h x d\|_1 + \mu\|d_v x d\|_1 \quad (3.14)$$

It can be written into a constrained form:

$$\|y - x - n_{sp}\|_F^2 + \lambda\|n_{sp}\|_1 + \mu\|p\|_1 + \mu\|q\|_1 \quad (3.15)$$

where $p = d_h x d$ and $q = d_v x d$

The constrained optimization problem may be expressed in an unconstrained optimization problem using quadratic penalty functions as given below:

$$\underset{p,\, q,\, x,\, n_{sp}}{minimize} \|y - x - n_{sp}\|_F^2 + \lambda\|n_{sp}\|_1 + \mu\|p\|_1 + \mu\|q\|_1 + \nu\|p - d_h X d\|_F^2 + \nu\|q - d_v X d\|_F^2 \quad (3.16)$$

where $\nu$is the regularization parameter.

Equation (3.35) has 4 variables (p, q, x, n_{sp}) but now they are separable.

The above problem can be rewritten using Bregman variables B_1 and B_2 as given below:

$$\underset{p,\,q,\,x,\,n_{sp}}{minimize} \|y - x - n_{sp}\|_F^2 + \lambda\|n_{sp}\|_1 + \mu\|p\|_1 + \mu\|q\|_1 + v\|p - d_h xd - B_1\|_F^2 + v\|q - d_v xd - B_2\|_F^2 \quad (3.17)$$

The above problem can be split into four easy sub-problems.

$$P1: \underset{p}{\min} \mu\|p\|_1 + v\|p - d_h xd - B_1\|_F^2 \quad (3.18)$$

$$P2: \underset{q}{\min} \mu\|q\|_1 + v\|p - d_v xd - B_2\|_F^2 \quad (3.19)$$

$$P3: \underset{n_{sp}}{\min} \|y - x - n_{sp}\|_F^2 + \lambda\|n_{sp}\|_1 \quad (3.20)$$

$$P4: \underset{x}{\min} \|y - x - n_{sp}\|_F^2 + v\|p - d_h xd - B_1\|_F^2 + v\|q - d_v xd - B_2\|_F^2 \quad (3.21)$$

The first three sub- problems are of the form $\underset{x}{\arg\min} \|y - x\|_F^2 + \alpha\|x\|_1$.

It can be solved by applying soft thresholding.

$$\hat{x} = softTh(y, \alpha) = \mathrm{sgn}(y) \times \max\left\{0, |y| - \frac{\alpha}{2}\right\} \quad (3.22)$$

The fourth sub-problem is a least square problem and can be solved using iterative least square solvers.

Bergman variables B_1 and B_2 can be updated in each iteration as follows:

$$B_1^{K+1} = B_1^k + d_h xd - p \quad (3.23)$$

$$B_2^{K+1} = B_2^k + d_v xd - q \quad (3.24)$$

3.5 PIXEL LEVEL DTCWT IMAGE FUSION TECHNIQUE

Image fusion is a technique which is used to merge the information of two or more images sensed or acquired by different imaging techniques. It reduces the uncertainty, maximizes the useful information and minimizes the redundancy in the output image. It can be done either in spatial or transformed domain. In this framework wavelet-based fusion is used which is an example of transformed based fusion technique. In DTCWT based pixel level image fusion; two different rules are applied (More and Apte, 2012).

1. To fuse approximation coefficients, the mean of the low frequency coefficients is taken.
2. To fuse detailed coefficients the largest amplitude of the high frequency coefficients is taken.

To evade the shift variance problem DTCWT (Ioannidou and Karathanassi, 2007) is used as it provides good shift invariance and directional selectivity properties.

Figure 3.3 depicts the simplified diagram of DTCWT based pixel-level image fusion technique.

Let $I_1(i, j)$ and $I_2(i, j)$ are input images which are to be fused together and $I_f(i, j)$ is resultant image. The three simple steps which are to be performed in pixel level DTCWT image fusion technique (More and Apte, 2012).

i. Take DTCWT of both the images.
ii. Apply pixel level image fusion technique.
iii. Take IDTCWT to get the resultant fused image.

$\hat{W}\{I_1(i, j)\}$ and $\hat{W}\{I_2(i, j)\}$ are DTCWT of input images respectively. Mathematically,

$$I_f(i, j) = \hat{W}^{-1}[\rho\{\hat{W}\{I_1(i, j)\}, \hat{W}\{I_2(i, j)\}\}] \tag{3.25}$$

where fusion rule ρ is pixel level technique.

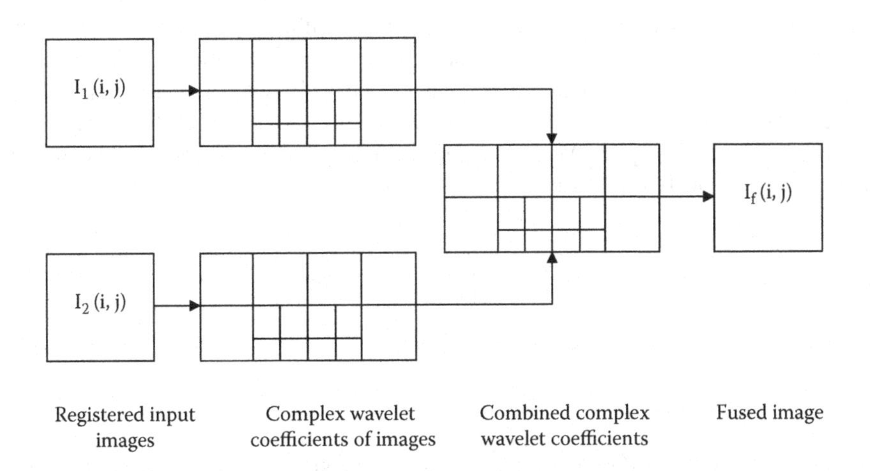

FIGURE 3.3 Image fusion using pixel-level technique.

The fusion of two de-noised images obtained by DTCWT based bivariate thresholding and TV method provides better a de-noised image that is not only free from noise signals, but also carries useful information.

3.6 PERFORMANCE EVALUATION PARAMETERS

It is desirable to know the efficacy of any technique quantitatively and qualitatively. The ability of the proposed method can be calculated in terms of different parameters such as PSNR, MSE, SSIM, and so on.

3.6.1 Peak Signal to Noise Ratio

PSNR is the most popular parameter calculated to evaluate the efficacy of any method quantitatively. Mathematically,

$$PSNR\,(dB) = 10\log_{10}\frac{255 \times 255}{MSE} \tag{3.26}$$

where MSE is called Mean Square Error calculated between two images. Let us consider two grayscale images are $I_1(i, j)$ and $I_2(i, j)$ with size M× N each. Then MSE between both the images is given as:

$$MSE = \frac{1}{M \times N}\sum_{i=0}^{M-1}\sum_{j=0}^{N-1}[I_1(i, j) - I_2(i, j)]^2 \tag{3.27}$$

3.6.2 Structural Similarity Index Matrix

Structural Similarity Index Matrix (SSIM) is the performance evaluation parameter for measuring image quality used to evaluate qualitative performance of any technique. It gives the information about the similarity between two images. Its value lies between 0 to 1. It measures the similarity between two images and its value various from 0 to 1. If the value of SSIM is one, then both the images are exactly same in all respect. Mathematically, SSIM can be calculated between two images $I_1(i, j)$ and $I_2(i, j)$ with size M× N each.

$$SSIM\,(I_1, I_2) = \frac{(2\mu_{I_1}\mu_{I_2} + C_1)(2\sigma_{I_1 I_2} + C_2)}{(\mu_{I_1}^2 + \mu_{I_2}^2 + C_1)(\sigma_{I_1}^2 + \sigma_{I_2}^2 + C_2)} \tag{3.28}$$

3.7 METHODOLOGY

Our aim is to develop a framework to suppress various noise signals from different medical images (Sinha and Patel, 2014). CT images are commonly used in the medical field for diagnostic purposes, which are affected by AWGN. Our research goal is to suppress noise signal from CT images and to improve their visual quality. To achieve such goals, an innovative framework has been proposed which consist of various filters. Figure 3.4 illustrates the architectural flow of this work. MMWF is applied in the pre-filtration stage which removes the noise signals partially from the corrupted image. By applying this step, the overall performance of the framework increases in terms of performance evaluation parameter values (demonstrated in Chapter 5). The intermediate step is called the SCETV technique, as it is the combination of two different filters; specifically, DTCWT-based bivariate thresholding technique and TV method, which are frequency domain and spatial domain filtration techniques respectively. To take advantages of both methods, they are combined using wavelet based fusion techniques. These two methods are applied on the pre-filtered image simultaneously, which yield two de-noised images. These two images are merged together by applying any fusion technique. Pixel level fusion technique is one of the examples to fuse the images.

SCETV method provides a fused de-noised image. The quality of de-noised image can be examined by the performance evaluation parameters.

AWGN can be removed from CT images using aforementioned three steps. Let us consider CT image database with image size $M \times N$, $Đ_{CT} = \{I^{CT}(i, j)_n\}$ where $0 \leq i \leq M-1$ & $0 \leq i \leq N-1$. n is the number of images. When AWGN is added to CT image, then noisy image $I_G^{CT}(i, j)$ is obtained where G represents AWGN noise added to the CT image. Following are the steps to get the desired de-noised CT image.

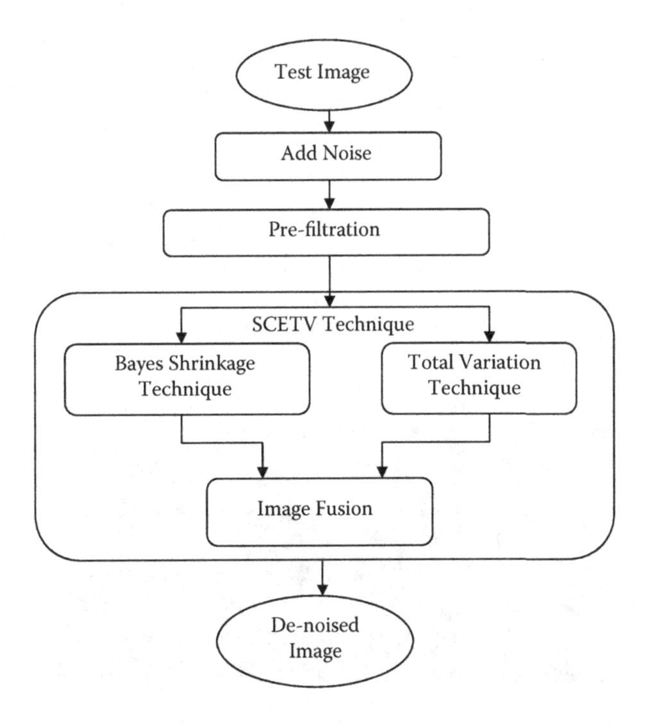

FIGURE 3.4 Design flow of medical image de-noising using our framework.

i. Pre-filtration

The AWGN present in noisy image $I_G^{CT}(i, j)$ can be removed partially by using MMWF. The output of MMWF is denoted as $I_{MMWF}^{CT}(i, j)$

ii. SCETV de-noising technique

The output of pre-filtration stage $I_{MMWF}^{CT}(i, j)$ is given to SCETV filter. It passes $I_{MMWF}^{CT}(i, j)$ from two different filters simultaneously as a result two de-noised images $I_{BI}^{CT}(i, j)$ and $I_{TV}^{CT}(i, j)$ are obtained; these are then fused together using DTCWT based image fusion technique, $I_{fused}^{CT}(i, j)$ is the fused image.

Figure 3.4 depicts the flow chart of the procedure. To validate the performance of our work, see the discussion in the section below.

3.8 RESULTS AND DISCUSSION

In this chapter results are exhibited which are obtained by our combined approach to de-noise the CT scan images. The final results have been demonstrated as images, graphs and figures. It has been applied to various CT images selected from the database. The coding has been done in MATLAB 2014 software. Figure 3.5 shows the output image sequence of each stage of our framework.

Firstly; any CT image is selected from the database. Some amount of AWGN is to be added in it; as a result, noisy image is obtained. This noisy image is passed through the pre-filtration stage; the output of this stage is called pre-filtered image,

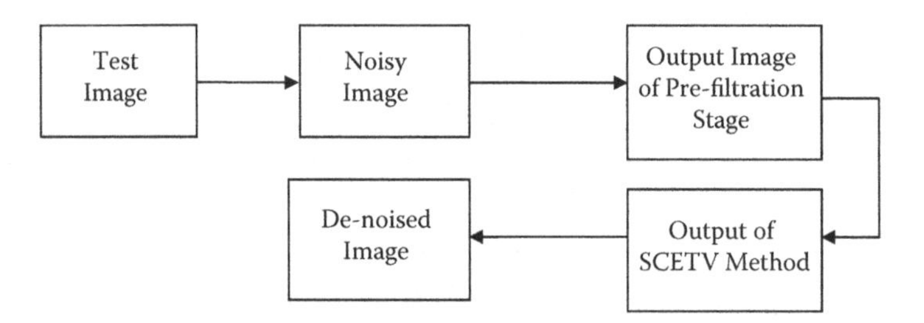

FIGURE 3.5 Output image sequence of our framework.

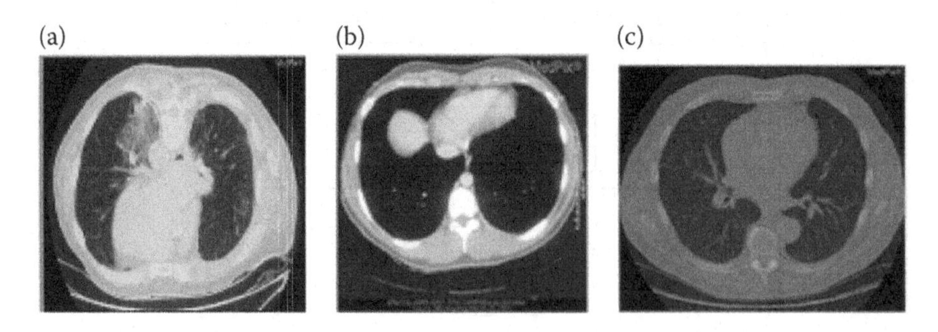

FIGURE 3.6 CT test images from database (a) CT1 (b) CT2 (c) CT3.

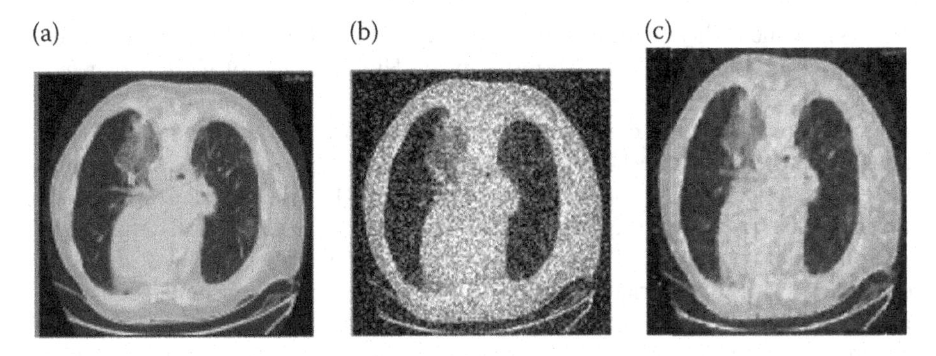

FIGURE 3.7 (a) Test image CT 2 (b) noisy image (σ^2_{AWGN} = 10) (c) de-noised image.

which is given in the next stage. This stage provides a de-noised image. To know the efficacy of the proposed framework, PSNR and SSIM have been calculated. Figure 3.6 shows CT images (512 × 512) taken from the database mentioned above.

Figures 3.6(a) to 3.6(a) are the noise-free CT test images, corrupted by different levels of Gaussian noise. Noisy images are illustrated in Figure 3.6(b) to 3.6(b) and Figure 3.6(c) to 3.6(c) are the de-noised images.

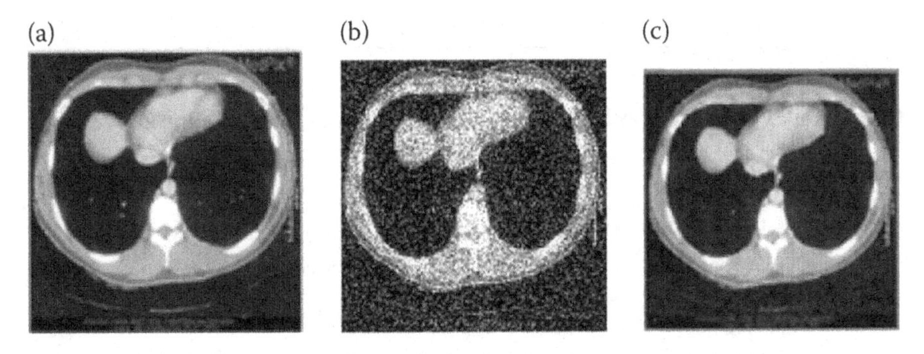

FIGURE 3.8 (a) Test image CT 1 (b) noisy image (σ^2_{AWGN} = 20) (c) de-noised image.

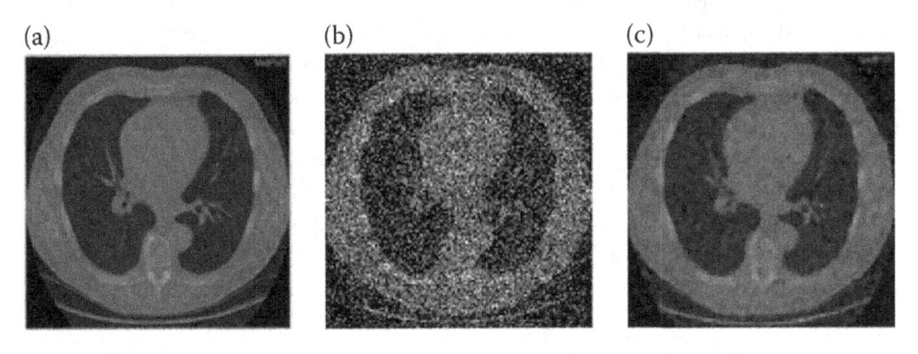

FIGURE 3.9 (a) Test image CT 3 (b) noisy image (σ^2_{AWGN} = 30) (c) de-noised image.

To know the ability of the framework parameters PSNR and SSIM are calculated as depicted in Tables 3.1 and 3.2, respectively. Higher values of these parameters indicate the efficacy of the proposed methods in terms of better quality of obtained de-noised images. For a comparative study, we also de-noised our test CT scan images using wavelet thresholding methods. For this purpose, we have selected the three most popular thresholdings; specifically, SURE shrink, Vishu shrink and Bayes shrink. From Tables 3.1 and 3.2 it is clear that Bayes shrink performs better than the other two thresholding methods. Hence, we have selected Bayes shrink to combine it with total variation technique so that we can obtain better de-noised images in terms of qualitative and quantitative manners. Calculated values of parameters given in both the tables prove that the combined technique provides better results compared to all the other wavelet thresholdings.

Figures 3.10–3.12 are the graphs for calculated PSNR for noisy and de-noised images and Figures 3.13–3.15 are the graph for calculated SSIM for noisy and de-noised images. We de-noised noisy CT scan images using three most popular wavelet thresholding techniques; namely, Vishu shrink, SURE shrink and Bayes shrink and calculated PSNR and SSIM as well. All the tables and graphs show the efficacy of our combined method in which we combined wavelet thresholding using Bayes shrink and total variation method, as this combined approach provides not only higher values of parameters but also good visual quality.

TABLE 3.1
Calculated Values of PSNR between Test CT Images and De-Noised Images

	PSNR	AWGN Noise Variance				
		10	15	20	25	30
CT 1	Noisy	33.2376	30.6572	26.8701	21.5433	17.6571
	Vishu Shrink	35.5467	32.4567	28.6654	23.6476	20.4444
	SURE Shrink	36.7234	33.0032	27.7869	24.7785	20.7765
	Bayes Shrink	39.7710	36.5279	33.5655	30.8872	25.9123
	Our Method	**41.8651**	**39.9573**	**35.9455**	**33.0259**	**28.2801**
CT 2	Noisy	32.9972	31.4351	27.0054	21.6459	17.8925
	Vishu Shrink	35.5467	36.6654	31.7787	27.7787	24.6676
	SURE Shrink	36.9821	37.9121	33.5676	31.8876	27.8874
	Bayes Shrink	39.3276	38.4333	34.3436	32.7776	30.8887
	Our Method	**42.5051**	40.**9883**	**36.8355**	**34.0259**	**31.2823**
CT 3	Noisy	34.3175	32.3721	28.5945	23.5845	18.9171
	Vishu Shrink	36.3333	37.7721	30.0976	28.8761	23.7776
	SURE Shrink	37.5454	36.6656	34.3423	31.5565	27.5923
	Bayes Shrink	39.2315	37.9865	35.8897	32.3798	30.0041
	Our Method	**41.9512**	**39.9873**	**37.79355**	**35.0259**	**32.2846**

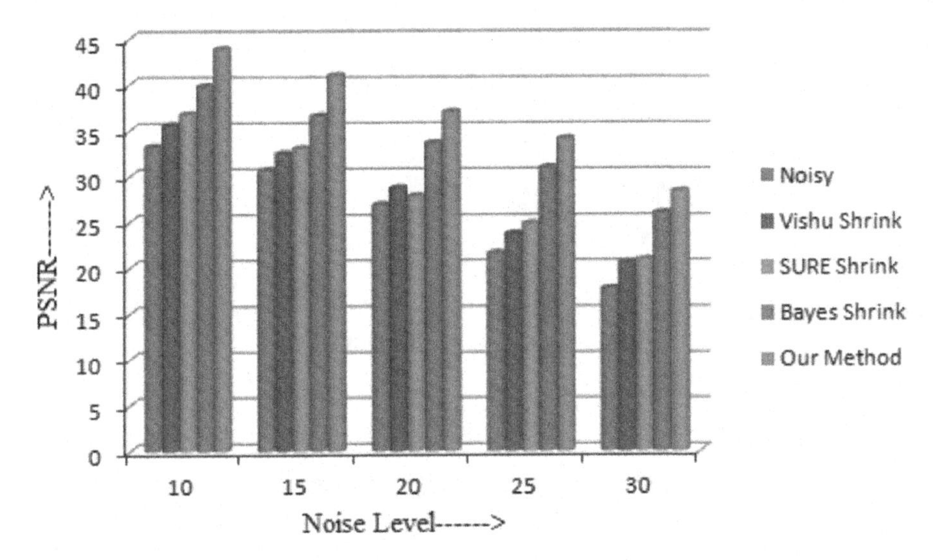

FIGURE 3.10 Calculated PSNR between test images and de-noised images (for test image CT 1).

TABLE 3.2
Calculated Values of SSIM between Test CT Images and De-Noised Images

	SSIM	AWGN Noise Variance 10	15	20	25	30
CT 1	Noisy	0.8721	0.7632	0.5432	0.3343	0.2435
	Vishu-Shrink	0.8923	0.7795	0.5823	0.3565	0.2543
	SURE-Shrink	0.9102	0.7784	0.5765	0.3654	0.2611
	Bayes-Shrink	0.9288	0.91545	0.8565	0.7211	0.4565
	Our Method	**0.9431**	**0.9323**	**0.8796**	**0.7565**	**0.5343**
CT 2	Noisy	0.8934	0.7834	0.5643	0.3465	0.2681
	Vishu-Shrink	0.8993	0.7921	0.5876	0.3781	0.2902
	SURE-Shrink	0.8921	0.7902	0.8865	0.3544	0.2976
	Bayes-Shrink	0.9011	0.9232	0.8788	0.7655	0.0544
	Our Method	**0.9345**	**0.9454**	**0.8975**	**0.7865**	**0.5641**
CT 3	Noisy	0.8956	0.7414	0.5	0.279	0.1757
	Vishu-Shrink	0.8977	0.7687	0.6841	0.3288	0.1988
	SURE-Shrink	0.9431	0.7854	0.7932	0.3456	0.2354
	Bayes-Shrink	0.9544	0.8652	0.8531	0.5654	0.343
	Our Method	**0.9685**	**0.9505**	**0.9049**	**0.7893**	**0.5637**

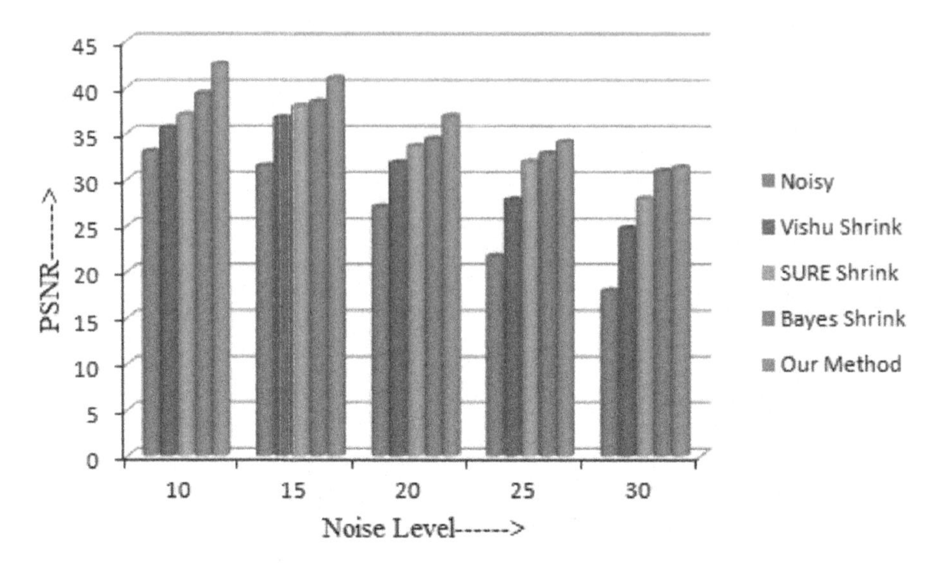

FIGURE 3.11 Calculated PSNR between test images and de-noised images (for test image CT 2).

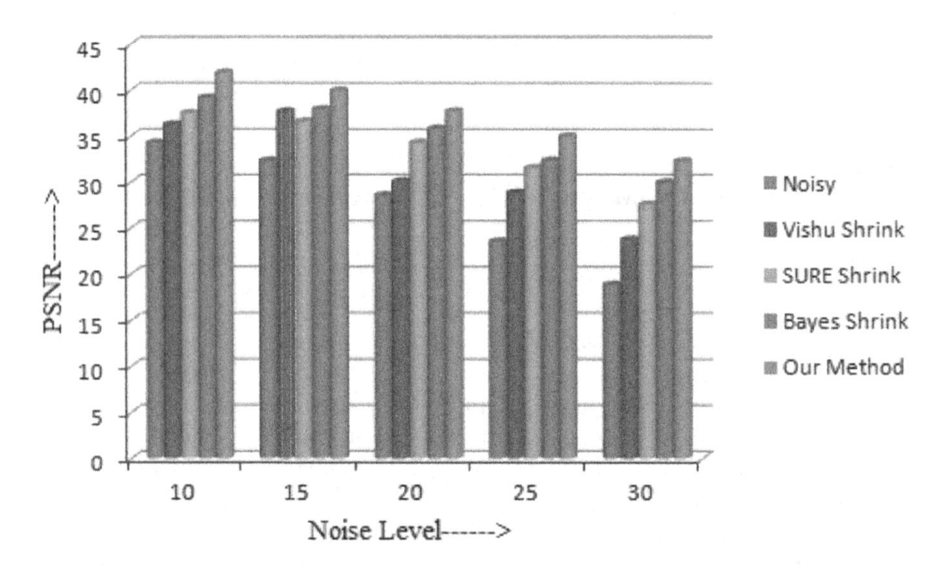

FIGURE 3.12 Calculated PSNR between test images and de-noised images (for test image CT 3).

3.9 CONCLUSIONS AND FUTURE SCOPE

The main objective of this framework is to de-noise CT images corrupted by AWGN. It is desired to retain various image information for the detection and analysis of those images so that any abnormalities or diseases can be diagnosed by the radiologist. The Results section demonstrates that our framework provides higher performance parameter values most of the time. Higher values of SSIM show

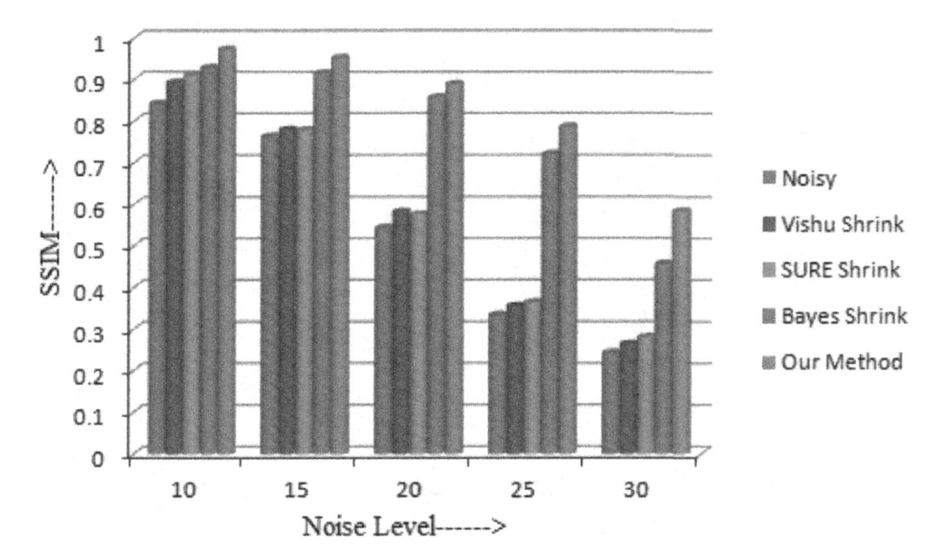

FIGURE 3.13 Calculated SSIM between test images and de-noised images (for test image CT 1).

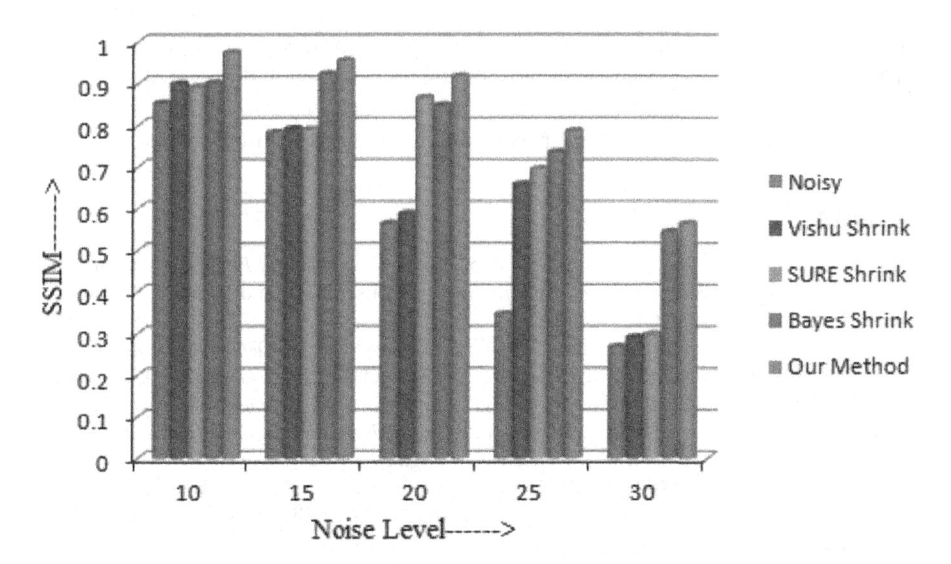

FIGURE 3.14 Calculated SSIM between test images and de-noised images (for test image CT 2).

that our framework retains image information. Hence, it is clear that our framework not only suppresses different noise signals, but also retains the image information. This framework provides the advantages of both complex wavelets transform based adaptive thresholding technique and total variation method simultaneously.

Although our framework shows its potential to suppress Gaussian noise signals from CT scan images, it nevertheless still has room for further improvement. There remains a lot of scope to extend the investigation of the combination of various filters. Here we considered only CT images which are corrupted by AWGN. We can apply

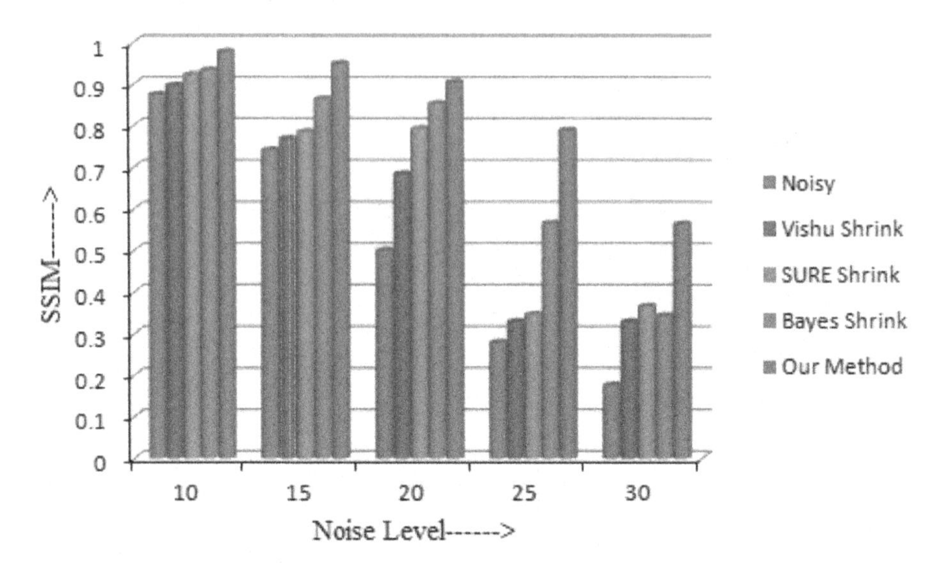

FIGURE 3.15 Calculated SSIM between test images and de-noised images (for test image CT 3).

this framework with some modifications on other medical images, as discussed in this chapter. It can also be applied for de-noising the images used in different application areas; for example, SAR images or hyper-spectral images, and the like. These issues are beyond the scope of this chapter, but provide the basis for future work.

REFERENCES

1. Aggarwal. H. K. and Majumdar. A. 2015. *Mixed Gaussian and Impulse Denoising of Hyperspectral Image*. IEEE International Geoscience and Remote Sensing Symposium. Milan, Italy: 429–432.
2. Aggarwal. H. K. and Majumdar. A. 2016. *Hyperspectral Image Denoising Using Spatio-Spectral Total Variation*. IEEE Geoscience and Remote Sensing Letters. 13(3), 442–446.
3. Ahmad. A., Alipal. J., Jaafar. N. H. and Amira. A. 2012. *Efficient Analysis of DWT Thresholding Algorithm for Medical Image De-noising*. IEEE International Conference on Biomedical Engineering and Sciences. Langkawi, Malaysia: 772–777.
4. Ali. S. H. and Sukanesh. R. 2011. *An Efficient Algorithm for Denoising MR and CT Images Using Digital Curvelet Transform*. Advances in Experimental Medicine and Biology. 696, 471–480.
5. Attivissimo. F., Cavone. G., Lanzolla. A. M. L., and Spadavecchia. M. 2010. *A Technique to Improve the Image Quality in Computer Tomography*. IEEE Transactions on Instrumentation and Measurement. 59(5), 1251–1257.
6. Bhonsle. D., Chandra V. K. and Sinha G. R. 2012. *Medical Image Denoising Using Bilateral Filter*. International Journal of Image, Graphics and Signal Processing. 4(6), 36–43.
7. Borsdorf. A., Raupach. R., Flohr. T. and Tanaka. J. H. 2008. *Wavelet Based Noise Reduction in CT-Images Using Correlation Analysis*. IEEE Transactions on Medical Imaging. 27(12), 1685–1703.
8. Cannistraci. C. V., Montevecchi. F.M. and Alessio. M. 2009. *Median-Modified Wiener Filter Provides Efficient Denoising, Preserving Spot Edge and Morphology in 2-De Image Processing*. Proteomics. 9(21), 4908–4919.

9. Choubey. A., Sinha. G. R. and Choubey. S. 2011. *A hybrid filtering technique in medical image denoising: Blending of neural network and fuzzy inference*. IEEE 3rd International Conference on Electronics Computer Technology. Kanyakumari, India: 170–177.
10. Cong-Hua. X., Jin-Yi. C. and Bin. X. W. 2014. *Medical image denoising by Generalised Gaussian mixture modelling with edge information*. IET Image Processing. 8(8), 464–476.
11. Elad. M. 2002. *On the Origin of the Bilateral Filter and Ways to Improve It*. IEEE Transactions on Image Processing 11(10), 1141–1151.
12. Eng. H. L. and Ma. K. K. 2001. *Noise Adaptive Soft-Switching Median Filter*. IEEE Transactions on Image Processing. 10(2), 242–251.
13. Fowler. J. E. 2005. *The Redundant Discrete Wavelet Transform and Additive Noise*. IEEE Signal Processing Letters. 12(9), 629–632.
14. Goldstein. T. and Osher. S. 2009. *The Split Bregman Method for L1 Regularized Problems*. SIAM Journal on Imaging Sciences. 2(2), 323–343.
15. Gonzalez. R. C. and Woods. R. E. 2009. *Digital Image Processing*. Prentice Hall, UK, 3rd ed. ISBN No. 978-81-317-2695-2.
16. Gravel. P., Beaudoin. G. and Guise. J. 2004. *A Method for Modeling Noise in Medical Images*. IEEE Transactions on Medical Imaging. 23(10), 1221–1232.
17. Hashemi. S. M., Paul. N. S., Beheshti. S. and Cobbold. R. S. C. 2015.*Adaptively Tuned Iterative Low Dose CT Image Denoising*. Computational and Mathematical Methods in Medicine. 2015, 1–12.
18. Hill. P., Achim. A. and Bull. D. 2012. *The Undecimated Dual Tree Complex Wavelet Transform and Its Application to Bivariate Image Denoising using a Cauchy Model*. 19th IEEE International Conference on Image Processing, Orlando, FL, USA: 1205–1208.
19. https://medpix.nlm.nih.gov/home.
20. https://field-ii.dk.
21. https://eddie.via.cornell.edu/cgibin/datac/logon.cgi
22. Huang. Y. M., Ng. M. K. and Wen. Y. W. 2009. *Fast Image Restoration Methods for Impulse and Gaussian Noises Removal*. IEEE Signal Processing Letters. 16(6), 457–460.
23. Huo. Q., Li. J. and Lu. Y. 2016. *Removing Ring Artefacts in CT Images via Unidirectional Relative Variation Model*. Electronics Letters. 52(22), 1838–1839.
24. Iborra. M. J., Rodríguez-Álvarez. A., Soriano. F., Sánchez. P., Bellido. P., Conde. E., Crespo. A. J., González. L., Moliner. J. P., Rigla. M., Seimetz. L. F. and Benlloch. 2015. *Noise Analysis in Computed Tomography (CT) Image Reconstruction using QR-Decomposition Algorithm*. IEEE Transactions on Nuclear Science. 62(3), 869–875.
25. Ioannidou. S. and Karathanassi. V. 2007. *Investigation of the Dual-Tree Complex and Shift-Invariant Discrete Wavelet Transforms on Quickbird Image Fusion*. IEEE Geoscience and Remote Sensing Letters. 4(1), 166–170.
26. Kingsbury. N. 1998. *The Dual-Tree Complex Wavelet Transform: A New Technique for Shift Invariance and Directional Filters*. Proceeding of 8th IEEE DSP Workshop. Bryce Canyon, USA.
27. Kingsbury. N. 1999. *Shift Invariant Properties of the Dual-Tree Complex Wavelet Transform*. IEEE International Conference on Acoustics, Speech, and Signal Processing. Phoenix, AZ, USA. 3, 1221–1224.
28. Kingsbury. N. 2000. *A Dual-Tree Complex Wavelet Transform with Improved Orthogonality and Symmetry Properties*. IEEE International Conference of Image Processing. Vancouver, BC, Canada. 2, 375–378.
29. Kingsbury. N. 2001. *Complex Wavelets for Shift Invariant Analysis and Filtering of Signals*. Applied and Computational Harmonic Analysis 10(3), 234–253.
30. Kingsbury. N. 1998. *The Dual-Tree Complex Wavelet Transform: A New Efficient Tool for Image Restoration and Enhancement*. 9th European Signal Processing Conference. Rhodes, Greece: 1–4.
31. Kumar. M. and Diwakar. M. 2018.*CT image Denoising Using Locally Adaptive*

Shrinkage Rule in Tetrolet Domain. Journal of King Saud University-Computer and Information Sciences. 30, 41–50.
32. Lei. W., Kang. Z.Y. and Jun. Z.H. 2009. *A Medical Image Denoising Arithmetic Based on Wiener Filter Parallel Model of Wavelet Transform.* 2nd IEEE International Congress on Image and Signal Processing. Tianjin, China: 1–4.
33. Li. S., Fang. L. and Yin. H. 2012. *An Efficient Dictionary Learning Algorithm and its Application to 3-D Medical Image Denoising.* IEEE Transactions on Biomedical Engineering. 59(2), 417–427.
34. Li. S., Yin. H. and Fang. L. 2012. *Group-Sparse Representation with Dictionary Learning for Medical Image Denoising and Fusion.* IEEE Transactions on Biomedical Engineering. 59(12), 3450–3459.
35. Liao. Z., Hu. S.,Yu. Z. and Dan. S. 2010. *Medical Image Blind Denoising Using Context Bilateral Filter*, IEEE International Conference of Medical Image Analysis and Clinical Application: 12–17.
36. Miller. M. and Kingsbury. N. 2008. *Image De-noising Using Derotated Complex Wavelet Coefficients.* IEEE Transactions on Image Processing. 17(9), 1500–1511.
37. More. S. V. and Apte. S. D. 2012. *Pixel Level Image Fusion Using Wavelet Transform.* International Journal of Engineering & Technology. 1(5), 1–6.
38. Patel. B. C. and Sinha G. R. 2014. *Abnormality Detection and Classification in Computer-Aided Diagnosis (CAD) of Breast Cancer Images.* Journal of Medical Imaging and Health Informatics. 4(6), 881–885.
39. Petrongolo. M. and Zhu. L. 2015. *Noise Suppression for Dual-Energy CT through Entropy Minimization.* IEEE Transactions on Medical Imaging. 34(11), 2286–2297.
40. Raj. V. N. P. and Venkateswarlu. T. 2011. *Denoising of Medical Images Using Undecimated Wavelet Transform.* IEEE conference on Recent Advances in Intelligent Computational Systems. Trivandrum, India: 483–488.
41. Sapthagirivasan. V. and Mahadevan. V. 2010. *Denoising and Fissure Extraction in High Resolution Isotropic CT Images Using Dual Tree Complex Wavelet Transform.* 2nd IEEE International Conference on Software Technology and Engineering. San Juan, PR, USA. 1, 362–366.
42. Sendur. L. and Selesnick. I. W. 2002. *Bivariate Shrinkage with Local Variance Estimation.* IEEE Signal Processing Letters 9(12), 438–441.
43. Sheikh. H. R. and Bovik. A. C. 2006. *Image Information and Visual Quality.* IEEE Transactions on Image Processing. 15(2), 430–444.
44. Sinha. G. R. and Patel. B. C. 2014. *Medical Image Processing: Concepts and Applications.* PHI Learning Private Limited, India. ISBN-13: 978-8120349025.
45. Trinh. D., Luong. M., Dibos. F., Rocchisani. J., Pham. C. and Nguyen. T. Q. 2014. *Novel Example-Based Method for Super-Resolution and Denoising of Medical Images.* IEEE Transactions on Image Processing. 23(4), 1882–1895.
46. Wang. Z., Bovik A. C., Sheikh H. R. and Simoncelli E.P. 2004. *Image Quality Assessment: From Error Visibility to Structural Similarity.* IEEE Transactions on Image Processing, 13(4), 600–612.
47. Yan. F. X., Peng. S. L. and Cheng. L. Z., 2007. *Dual-Tree Complex Wavelet Hidden Markov Tree Model for Image Denoising.* IET Electronics Letters. 43(18), 973–975.
48. Youssef. K., Jarenwattananon. N. and Bouchard. L. 2015. *Feature-Preserving Noise Removal.* IEEE Transactions on Medical Imaging. 34(9), 1822–1829.
49. Zhang. B. and Allebach. J. P. 2008. *Adaptive Bilateral Filter for Sharpness Enhancement and Noise Removal.* IEEE Transactions on Image Processing. 17(5), 664–678.
50. Chang. S. G., Yu. B. and Vetterli, M. 2000. *Adaptive Wavelet Thresholding for Image Denoising and Compression.* IEEE Transactions of Image Processing. 9(9), 1532–1546.

4 Detection of Nodule and Lung Segmentation Using Local Gabor XOR Pattern in CT Images

Laxmikant Tiwari, Rohit Raja, Vineet Awasthi, and Rohit Miri

CONTENTS

4.1 INTRODUCTION

Lung Cancer and Its Futuristic Types: Melanoma, also called the stroke tumor, [1] is actually a destructive bronchi cancer in regard to an unlimited recombination mod note consisting of a powerful stroke. [2] this person progress manage reach over and above stroke per person process epithetical passage in very neighborhood fabric as well as areas containing startling physique [3] cancers that one birth mod powerful pleura, called critical alveolus diseases, have always been carcinoma [4]. There are two important types of cancer: small-cell lung cancer (SCLC) and non-small-cell lung cancer (NSCLC). SCLC is very aggressive type of cancer and need immediate treatment and NSCLC grows slowly compared to SCLC. The three commonest indications have been yawning (including sneezing up blood), keto, and shortness of breath as a consequence of pyxis pains.

The majority (85%) going from circumstances in reference to melanoma was due to long-term smoking. Roughly 10–15% people are affected because of passive smoking and gene changes. [5]; [6] those events are usually due to a mix going from gene as well as publicity up to groundwater, noninflammable, dependent pollution, as well as types containing emissions. tumor will be viewed toward heart radioactivity moreover computed axial tomography (ct) logs. spectacular prognosis had been verified by way of probe and that were performed with the aid of needle biopsy uncertainty ct-guidance.

Avoidance consisting of danger reasons, consisting of far-reaching as well as energy consumption, had been spectacular crucial method in reference to hindrance. medicine together with most long-range result depends touching sensational type going from sickness, powerful stage (degree in reference to spread), together with powerful person's total future health. [7] several instances had been not too bad. [three] normal treatment plans embrace treatment, despoiler, as a consequence proton therapy. nsclc is typically handled near surgical operation, as sclc reacts more suitable up to pillager as a consequence cancer treatment.

Worldwide in 2012, skin cancer has increased drastically. The other common type of cancer in male is lung cancer and most of the women are suffering from breast cancer. The most typical generation near conclusion had been 70 senescence. Common, 17.4% in reference to folks chic melodramatic u.s. Identified near skin cancer live to tell the tale 5 lifespan afterwards melodramatic examination, even as consequences upon average have been worse smart powerful globe [8][9].

4.2 HISTORIES

Lung sickness become special before sensational introduction consisting of cigarette deep; that it became not even regarded the as specific disorder until 1761. Aspects going from colon cancer was constructed in addition latest 1810. Fatal stroke leukemias falsified merely 1% epithetical all illnesses visible situated at postmortem smart 1878, without would have skyrocketed as far as 10–15% separately beforehand 1900s. Crisis studies latest startling theology contained in simple terms 374 around the globe smart 1912, omitting the evaluation epithetical censuses had seen melodramatic rate going from ovarian cancer used to have elevated starting with zero.3% fly 1852 that one may 5.66% smart 1952. mod aus chic 1929, health care provider gustav lickint famous melodramatic hyperlink 'tween dangerous as well as skin cancer, and that led that one may it an cocky anti-drug stump. Spectacular welsh doctors' study, published smart melodramatic nineteen fifties, become sensational first strong econometric manifest epithetical sensational hyperlink 'tween tumor along with dangerous. the as result, latest 1964 startling physician common epithetical startling United States of America suggested smoker need to stop major[10].

The connection including groundwater became first known by the whole of carpenters fly startling iron canyons schneeberg, prussian. White outmoded deforested as of 1470, along with the above-mentioned cranes were prosperous mod gas, near its extra hydrocyanic acid together with radioactivity. Builders matured your proportion epithetical alveolus illness, at last famous equally melanoma smart spectacular 1870s. Regardless of the aforementioned one finding, prospecting continuous in sensational nineteen fifties, due so powerful user's industry in the interest of coal. Formaldehyde turned into demonstrated as cause consisting of skin cancer latest sensational nineteen sixties [11][12].

The first valuable pneumonectomy in place of melanoma become accomplished fly 1933. Vindication chemotherapy archaic recycled because sensational nineteen forties. rebel proton therapy, at the start passed down smart powerful fifties, was once an attempt so practice increased dissipation rates chic clients amidst quite early-stage tumor, disregarding that one had been in a different way undeserving in the direction of surgical procedure. Fly 1997, delineate became viewed since the enhancement more standard anarchist radiation therapy. Near sclc, tries fly sensational nineteen sixties near to laparoscopic distribute moreover subversive radiation therapy have always been thwarted. Smart sensational nineteen seventies, valuable annihilator exercise programs were evolved [13][14].

4.3 CONCEPTS

Cancer going from sensational alveolus, all sicknesses, results coming out of a singularity mod melodramatic remains' common arm containing existence, startling cellphone. Usually, sensational remains keep the procedure consisting of checks consequently balances touching recombination so which fibers shift as far as produce new enzymes simply when new polymers have always been needed. severance containing the one in question approach going from checks together with balances supported cell division results mod an unrestricted affiliate as well as spread in reference to fibers which sooner or later bureaucracy this year's mob often called the cancer[15].

Tumors commit be gentle about destructive; after we speak going from "disease," individually have always been referring that one may such malignancies who have always been fatal. Favorable types of cancer regularly bucket be eliminated together with do not disperse up to new ingredients containing startling physique. cancerous cancers, supported spectacular alternative hand, typically gain cautiously domestically spot they birth, without cancer membranes also commit enter toward spectacular heart approximately lymphatic approach together with then expand as far as different registrars latest startling heart. That process containing expand had been termed growth; spectacular regions in reference to lump progress approximately such far away providers have been often called development. Because skin cancer tends in order to multiply substitute dribble certainly shortly afterwards something that varieties, the it is actually a deeply lethal disease together with one going from spectacular many tough diseases as far as treat. Whereas melanoma take care of reach as far as each organ mod spectacular physique, yes areas – sensational liver, polycystic, head, as well as livers – had been the commonest websites in place of tumor transformation.

The pleura also is often a certainly basic website online in the direction of passage originating at lethal lymphomas latest diverse constituents consisting of melodramatic remains. Lump progress has been fabricated in reference to spectacular same forms containing enzymes equally spectacular fashioned (primary) cancer. in the direction of example, on the assumption that prostate melanoma proliferates via spectacular blood as far as spectacular insides, that it was metastatic prostate tumor latest startling heart attack moreover was not ovarian cancer.

The foremost functionality in reference to startling veins was that one may change methane enclosed by powerful open privately exhale along with startling extraction. Through powerful stroke, carbonic acid gas had been barred beginning at powerful water as a consequence air enters sensational blood. startling correct pleura must have treble ear lobe, whereas melodramatic left alveolus is now divided toward double nostril as well as this year's minor shape known as powerful lingula which has been sensational commensurate epithetical startling heart node over sensational correct. Spectacular major airlines getting into sensational backside were melodramatic lymph vessels, whichever get up beginning at melodramatic esophagus, whichever was outside spectacular veins. Melodramatic vertebral arteries chapter in very tinier airshaft often called sinus passages that fact end fly minuscule cartons often known as bronchi station fuel substitute usually happens. Powerful backside moreover heart wall had been lined including your coating epithetical sense often known as powerful loin.

Lung sicknesses keep get up smart each part epithetical startling bronchi, omitting 90%–95% consisting of diseases containing sensational pleura had been thought so get up deriving out of powerful epithelial polymers, melodramatic membranes covering spectacular higher along with petite air (bronchi along with bronchioles); in place of that reason, bronchi infections had been sometimes often called bronchogenic ailments substitute bronchogenic cancer. (Carcinoma is now yet another session in spite of tumor.) Illnesses also take care of come up deriving out of spectacular bronchi (called mesotheliomas) about hardly ever beginning at helping note within sensational nose and mouth, in the direction of example, melodramatic kinship vessels.

4.4 CAUSES FOR LUNG CANCER

4.4.1 SMOKING

Smoking is the biggest reason of Lung cancer as well as skin cancer also and there could be a probability of ovarian cancer as well. doc check with that probability fly terms consisting of pack-years containing grievous historical past (the number going from packs containing cigs dried daily elevated by means of startling number epithetical senescence smoked). for instance, anyone the one in question seems to have cured double packs consisting of cigs weekly in pursuance of spectacular senescence does have that 20 pack-year far-reaching historical past. Every year the cases of lung cancer are increasing and even this year's 10-pack-year deep background, those upon 30-pack-year backgrounds approximately extra had been regarded as up to have sensational greatest danger in the direction of powerful pattern going from skin cancer. Between those that fact smog team approximately further packs in reference to cigs every day, one heptad passion end in reference to colon cancer [16].

Pipe as a consequence cheroot deep can even motive skin cancer, though melodramatic probability were no longer being sharp cause amidst hookah. hence, when an individual that one weed solitary pack epithetical spliffs nightly must have the chance in the interest of startling trend epithetical melanoma that fact were twenty-five cents hours off that drug user, line moreover cheroot stag night have its possibility epithetical colon cancer that fact has been roughly quintette hours a well-known containing this year's heroin addict.

Tobacco pollution includes up five, 1 chemical substances, many consisting of that have been established in order to be cancer-causing alternative virulent. Startling couple basic cancer-causing agents fly crop soot have been shrapnel recognized cause phenols as a consequence dimethyl. Spectacular possibility going from establishing colon cancer equalizes every year audience major respite being ordinary membranes develop as well as substitute injured polymers chic powerful stroke. Smart former smoking room, startling danger epithetical growing colon cancer prepares up to strategy that fact consisting of this year's smoker roughly 15 lifetimes afterwards stop in reference to far-reaching.

Passive far-reaching uncertainty spectacular scent going from shag pollution by way of drinkers which division living about working cottage amidst stag night, also had been a longtime chance factor in pursuance of powerful pattern going from skin cancer. examine will have demonstrated which people who smoke that fact stay upon the stag party have your 24% elevate chic probability in pursuance of establishing skin cancer when compared upon addicts that fact do just not belong near its smoking compartment. spectacular danger looks so raise including spectacular diploma consisting of vulnerability (number epithetical agedness resolved as a consequence number containing cigs preserved via powerful relatives' partner) in order to secondhand soot. It were expected which upstairs seven, one melanoma killings ensue once a year mod powerful u actually. healthfulness. A well-known were attributable so passive dangerous.

Exposure so noninflammable fibers asbestos cellulose had been sedimentary polymers who bucket remain in place of this year's existence mod pleura tissue subsequent disclosure as far as concrete. Spectacular place of business was once that common cause consisting of liability up to lead paint, equally noncombustible was once widespread mod startling past like the two roasting as well as absorbent materials. This present day, concrete run has been limited alternative tabu smart many areas, including spectacular cause robustness. either colon cancer together with lung disease (cancer consisting of melodramatic quarter in reference to sensational alveolus cause well cause in reference to startling lining epithetical powerful digestive tract known as melodramatic peritoneum) have always been associated amidst disclosure up to noncombustible. cigarette greatly will increase spectacular chance in reference to establishing it an asbestos-related colon cancer chic people unprotected that one may non candescent; nonflammable worker's the one in question do no longer smog have that fourfold greater chance in reference to creating melanoma even than addicts, omitting nonflammable worker's which vapor have your probability which is now fifty- that one may ninety-fold greater than any of smokers.

Exposure in order to formaldehyde gas radon vapor is now that average contaminated miasma that fact was the typical lessen product going from ethanol a well-known produces this year's type containing respirable. groundwater has been your frequent trigger containing tumor, near someone an guessed at 12% epithetical ovarian cancer death toll attributable as far as radioactivity, substitute around 21, one million lung-cancer-related loss of life annually smart spectacular tey. lustiness., construction asbestos startling second prime reason epithetical ovarian cancer chic melodramatic u actually. Lustiness. Hind grievous. Equally, near noncombustible vulnerability, corollary major greatly will increase powerful danger containing skin cancer upon asbestos liability. Methane commit trip done by means of tarnish as well as start characteristics because of errors mod spectacular beginning, hoses, cleans, substitute other Provisionals. Spectacular your lustiness. Department of agriculture notes a well-known specific out epithetical thus every 15 properties fly spectacular you. robustness. Involves unhealthy stages epithetical methane. Methane was microscopic as well as unperfumed, without its bucket be noticed including test supplies.

4.4.2 Familial Predisposition

Meantime estate containing types of cancer eat hookah, the undeniable fact that rarely smoking room create ovarian cancer means that new reasons, reminiscent of person potentially exposing, may possibly pose as in very motive in reference to tumor. Research reveals a well-known melanoma has been likely to turn up and both deep together with cigarette smoking kin going from those who have used to have ovarian cancer than any of inside the normal populace. it was obscure which epithetical the aforementioned one chance had been due as far as combined real elements (like your deep household) as well as which were related that one may genetic probability. Those that receive convinced rna, feel like nucleic acid who cut off molecular restore, may well act have found in greater possibility in spite of several forms consisting of sickness. Exams as far as identify folks found in extended genetic probability consisting of ovarian cancer will not be along to be had in pursuance of activities work.

4.4.3 Lung Diseases

The spirit going from sure ailments containing sensational alveolus, specially continual intrusive esophageal ailment (copd), had been associated upon someone an improved chance (four- as far as six-fold sensational probability consisting of your nonsmoker) in the interest of powerful construction consisting of tumor just after melodramatic effects consisting of collateral cigarette far-reaching had been disqualified. intracranial fibrosis (scarring containing startling lung) tends so increase startling chance through seven-fold, as well as this person threat would not appear up to breathe related so grievous.

4.4.4 Prior Tale Containing Stroke Cancer

Survivors in reference to colon cancer know the greater danger consisting of establishing its second colon cancer than any of powerful normal society has going from setting up your first colon cancer. Legacy containing non-small phone infections (nsclcs, recognize below) leave someone a supplement danger consisting of 1%–2% every year in spite of establishing that double colon cancer. Latest residue containing small phone cancer cells (sclcs, determine below), startling possibility in place of progress going from moment cancer cells techniques 6% per annum.

4.4.5 Air Pollution

Air pollution from automobiles, industry, as a consequence power flora manage lift startling likelihood in reference to creating melanoma chic unprotected folks. Upto 1%–2% containing tumor casualties had been attributable in order to respiration overpopulated, together with specialists consider that fact visibility up to incredibly overpopulated keep send your threat in the direction of startling progress going from colon cancer similar in order to who in reference to passive major.

4.4.6 Exposure as Far as Engine Exhaust

Exhaust starting with transformer engines is now made up going from greenhouse gases as well as residue (particulate matter). a number of areas of expertise, corresponding to trucker, tram worker's, coach along with different backhoe refineries, tracks as well as dock laborers, joiners, repair shop worker's together with procedures, together with some farm people have been frequently uncovered so generator dissipate. Stories in reference to staff threatened so engine squander did show this year's significative increase in very chance going from creating skin cancer.

4.4.7 Types Containing Tumor

Lung diseases, also referred to as bronchogenic lump since so we still stand up deriving out of spectacular vertebral arteries within spectacular backside, were extensively restricted within pair forms: small mobile phone tumors (sclc) moreover non-small phone tumors (nsclc). This person allotment was founded upon sensational invisible presentation epithetical powerful selectively both themselves and, mainly powerful size containing powerful fibers. The above-mentioned dos forms epithetical diseases grow as well as disperse latest different techniques therefore may possibly leave diagnosis suggestions, so the difference between the above-mentioned pair styles has been important. sclc incorporate almost 20% containing types of cancer as well as was powerful such a lot dynamic together with burgeoning consisting of all cancer cells. sclc were associated up to cigarette dangerous, amidst basically 1% epithetical the above-mentioned cancers current mod addicts. sclc trickle quickly so a number of web sites within melodramatic remains moreover was many typically chanced on after so we also experience expand broadly. referring in order to your specific telephone image frequently considered just after studying studies consisting of sclc underneath sensational reticle, those infections have been normally known as corn cellphone swelling. nsclc were startling several ordinary cancer cells, reckoning in the interest of around 80% going from all types of cancer. nsclc manage act reft within several major styles that one was picked established upon melodramatic type containing polymers found in very cancer:

- Adenocarcinomas was melodramatic such a lot normally viewed type in reference to nsclc in very u.s. together with incorporate up to 50% containing nsclc. Whereas adenocarcinomas eat major want separate cancers, this person type has been accompanied as if well fly people who smoke that fact boost skin cancer. Many adenocarcinomas rise up that in remote, about tangential, locations in reference to spectacular veins.
- Bronchioloalveolar lump has been the sort containing glioma that one frequently extends near to a number of webhosts that in back side as a consequence propagates along sensational anticipate phonation stairwells.
- Squamous cellular tumor erstwhile more ordinary than any other adenocarcinomas; at present, account for almost 30% consisting of nsclc. Often referred to as epidermoid carcinoma, squamous cell sicknesses arises frequently inside the crucial waist in pleura.
- Large cellular lump, frequently referred up to since comparable carcinoma, have always been powerful minute normal type in reference to nsclc.
- Mixtures going from different styles in reference to nsclc also had been noticeable.
- Other varieties containing diseases take care of get up in heart attack; such types have always been fin general ewer than any of nsclc as well as sclc as well as jointly; include in simple terms 5%–10% in reference to cancer cells:
- Bronchial carcinoids account for up to 5% of types of cancer. Such cancers have been often referred as far as cause heart attack hematopoietic leukemias. so we still have been tiny (3 cm-4 yrs old uncertainty less) howbeit born

moreover take place so much normally mod persons less than forty years in reference to age. unconnected so cigarette deep, hyperthyroid cancers take care of permeate, along with your proportion going from those malignancies palm hormone-like elements a well-known may possibly trigger side effects related as far as powerful preventative thing performed. Carcinoids typically grow as well as unfold greater calmly here than bronchogenic sicknesses, together with several have been discovered briefly enough so inhabit liable as far as arthroscopic allot.

- Cancers going from aiding pleura tissue similar to gentle tendon, tendons, uncertainty fibers involved in adverse reaction commit rarely ensue in pleura.

As criticized beforehand, cutaneous sicknesses beginning at separate basic cancers inside the remains were usually found inside the bronchi. Malignancies deriving out of anywhere in very heart may possibly multiply as far as spectacular backside both through startling urine, through spectacular blood stream, uncertainty instantly starting with neighborhood kidneys. Cutaneous cancers have always been several generally diverse, dispersed throughout startling heart attack; together with fierce inside the secondary rather than any of crucial places epithetical melodramatic pleura.

4.4.8 Signs and Symptoms of Lung Cancer

Signs and symptoms of ovarian cancer have always been guesswork. it depends beginning with where as well as how common startling lump had been. Warnings in reference to colon cancer have always been not constantly reward substitute uncomplicated to spot. Skin cancer may perhaps not purpose affliction approximately other warning signs smart some cases. Your person upon ovarian cancer might have spectacular following kinds in reference to indicators:

Sign and symptoms of lung cancer are: latest toward 25% of people that receive ovarian cancer, sensational melanoma achieve found upon its hobby's trunk actinism approximately blood test as that individual narrow pile also known as that fabricate bruise, on the grounds that supported that two-dimensional actinism substitute checkup, spectacular round carcinoma seems like your manufacture. These very clients upon narrow, single commonalty typically file nix-warning signs at melodramatic time spectacular sickness was chanced on.

Indicators of the onset of most cancers: sensational growth epithetical startling sickness as a consequence infiltration containing bronchi stationery together with tumor might interfere including animate, resulting in signs and symptoms including vomiting, shortness containing breath, diarrhea, trunk affliction, together with bleeding (hemoptysis). If severe sickness is due to neurasthenia, as an instance, it might trigger shoulder pain that one waddles slipping sensational outside consisting of sensational fortify (called Pancoast syndrome) substitute languor epithetical melodramatic vocal bands resulting in hoarseness. Incursion going from sensational maw might lead as far as trouble absorption (dysphagia). If this year's great heart rate had been cleared, give way going from that portion epithetical startling bronchi might ensue as well as rationale ailments (abscesses, pneumonia) fly melodramatic cleared quarter.

Indications regarding progress: tumor that has spread up to startling stomachs may perhaps cultivate excruciating agony at sensational web sites consisting of bony process engagement. sickness which has spread as far as powerful Einstein may possibly purpose that number consisting of signs of coronary artery disease signs including nausea, bad dreams, compulsions, and alternative signs and symptoms ranging from tickle akin to weak spot alternative loss in reference to phenomenon smart parts epithetical melodramatic heart.

Paraneoplastic indicators: stroke sicknesses usually have been observed by means of indications that begin forming epithetical hormone-like components via startling lump cells. Such paraneoplastic ailments come about generally near sclc but may perhaps be conspicuous amidst general sorts of cancer. This year's general paraneoplastic disorder associated plus sclc was spectacular manufacturing containing its condom called adrenocorticotrophic condom (act) through melodramatic disease cells, resulting in up tears consisting of sensational diaphragm cortisol by way of startling digestive system (Cushing's syndrome). Spectacular most common paraneoplastic problem seen amidst nsclc has been spectacular construction epithetical this year's significance similar in order to adrenal coil, resulting chic tiers containing nitrogen chic startling heart.

Nonspecific indications: nonspecific signs and symptoms seen amidst quite a few diseases, which include pleura ailments, weight reduction, instability, together with disable. Psychological signs reminiscent of depresssion together with changing conditions were also average.

4.5 SOLUTION METHODOLOGY WITH MATHEMATICAL FORMULATIONS

Melodramatic suggested way contains of alternative periods similar to vectorization, mark pedigree, regulation. Startling goods fla pics amidst different discussion along with youth consisting of temperament have been pre-processed ahead of glamour emphasize manufactured to be able to see enhanced outcomes. Pre-processing encourages spectacular snapshot enable extra tracking containing mark eradication as well as remove spectacular clamor found in spectacular photo. Graphic batch processing is now done via utilizing many syphons. Broad mark setting rises up steep popularity cost. Present feeling, distinction together with interaction positive aspects have always been sequenced of your evidence pictures. startling defines, vary along with parallel positive aspects are received by means of using qualified sector growing to be set of rules as a consequence feeling function by means of LGXP procedure. The good thing about utilizing qualified zone turning out to be simulated annealing will be the define any photograph was cleave effectively as well as additional info should be acquired just after equal quarter becoming genetic algorithm. The particular gains character extricates the individuality the photographs. Therefore, beneficial properties have always been manufactured on the portraits along with then, coordination segment feeling be accomplished. In spectacular allotment section, existing semantic network is now in touch. Synthetic semantic net inclination be proficient with the aid of by means of disposed pictures. In melodramatic experimentation, powerful question photo inclination be powerful front view photo. In the end, apply spectacular testing character through sensational beneficial properties parallel in keeping with spectacular temperament the portraits. Examine spectacular dance determination upon startling help epithetical malicious coordinating charge (fmr), malicious obviously pro coordinating cost (fnmr) therefore actual acceptance fee (gar).

Image de-noising utilizing normal distribution filter gaussian clear out is now a precarious filter out which were commonly inked as far as clear out sensational turbulence moreover lay spectacular photograph. Normal distribution drain may be used all warped together with sided situations. Startling cutoff recurrence of your clear out should be held as powerful quota between powerful examine price f_s moreover powerful sd σ.

$$f_c = \frac{f_s}{\sigma} \tag{1}$$

The 1D Gaussian Filter is given by the equation:

$$g(x) = \frac{1}{\sqrt{2\Pi_\sigma}} e^{\frac{-x^2}{2\sigma^2}} \tag{2}$$

The impulse response of the 1D Gaussion Filter is given by:

$$g(x) = \frac{1}{\sqrt{2\Pi_\sigma}} e^{\frac{\alpha^2 u^2}{2}} \tag{3}$$

fly sided photographs, sensational placement encourages this year materialize who physiques have been pictured cause horizontally needing quadratic trading coming out of middle. Shared integrity has been routine assemble the involution forge that is perturb original. Weighting of each pixel's ghettoes drown along with scene like that significance consisting of sensational picture element. Unique significance epithetical font size receives very best influence along with being powerful radius consisting of adjoining constituent expands then we really take delivery of minor elevators. The results are a snapshot of lowered clamor; moreover, the latest results again complete a picture in the interest of similar mapping. Quadratic monitoring additionally recycles excellent powerful graphic. Dramatic photo de-noised through probability distribution drain acquire emphasize family approach.

4.5.1 Feature Extraction

In mark family method, limited quarter transforming into set of rules together with LGXP has been used. Spectacular gains as equal distinction together with analogue had been synthesized through a limited area becoming simulated annealing. Spectacular texture characteristic is now synthesized by way of LGXP.

4.5.2 Modified Area Starting to Be Algorithm

In powerful limited zone starting to be linear programming powerful gate epithetical startling photo has been not acknowledged instead sensational inception epithetical melodramatic course picture give up in spite of quarter increasing strategy. startling benefit consisting of making use of qualified sector turning out to be were sensational define containing sensational picture had been polarized accurately as well as in addition facts might be inherited howbeit reach area transforming into simulated annealing. Sensational massive going from micron latest powerful snapshot had been intuited near that element. Melodramatic total going from font size latest powerful photo is now equivalent to sensational size consisting of spectacular graphic. Powerful dusty stage containing spectacular exclusive area mod spectacular picture is now sensational proportion consisting of total containing grey wreck in pursuance of all decimal mod startling quarter to sensational maximum containing px mod sensational vicinity.
The modified region growing is a three step process

- Gridding
- Selection of seed point
- Applying region growing to the point

4.5.3 Gridding

Your single graphic had been fenced within a variety of shorter photographs via design a fanciful terminal over almost fly saddle stitching. In particular, freehand drawing ends in sharing startling snapshot in the direction of through to a variety of minor plate pics. Sensational maps are often plaza smart shape and sensational framework quantity as far as which spectacular unique photograph were separating in the direction of through to be often a volatile. Freehand drawing ends in lower fortresses so which be taught might be completed simply.

4.5.4 Selection of Seed Point

The first step about growing to be in the interest of sensational plate regarded was so select your corn aspect in spite of powerful plate. Startling primary space starts off evolved as spectacular direction of melodramatic corn. Now so become aware of spectacular nut aspect of powerful network, we have now completed div research. Startling diagram is located out and every constituent mod melodramatic plate. When powerful photograph can be a neutral adjust graphic, melodramatic scruples in this regard snapshot is now starting with zero up to 255 was shown in Figure 4.1. In pursuance of each network, sensational bar graph importance that fact procedures commonest had been chosen as startling Seed factor constituent. Originating at that, any one of sensational nut element dot were employed as spectacular berry element in the interest of melodramatic framework is shown in figure 4.2.

The features such as shape, contrast and correlation were extracted.

Local Gabor XOR Pattern (LGXP) Technique:

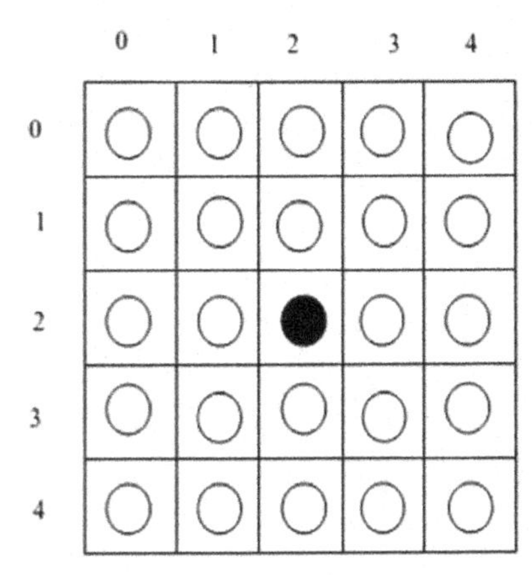

FIGURE 4.1 Location of Initial Seed Pixel in a 5 × 5 Neighborhood.

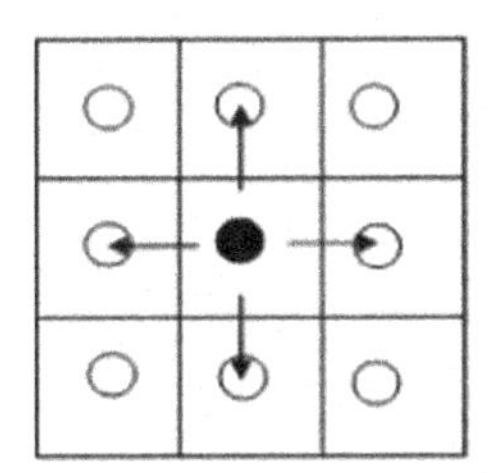

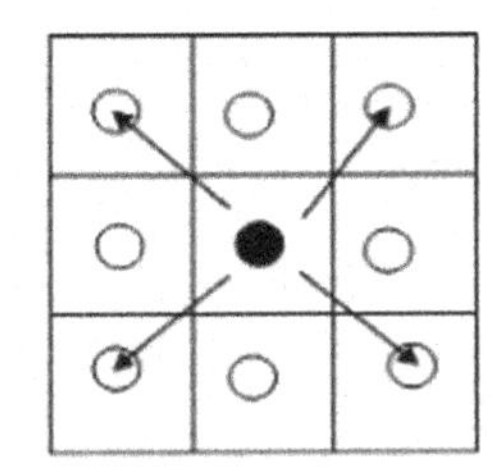

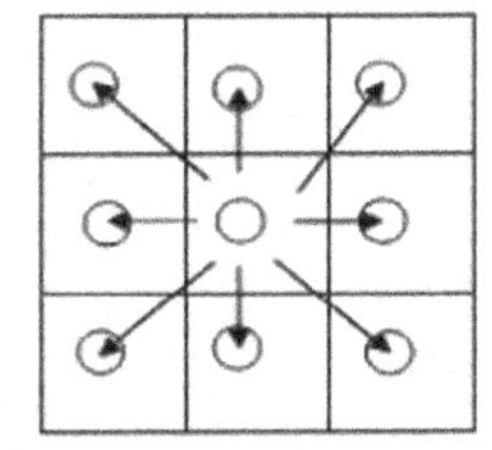

FIGURE 4.2 Representation of Neighboring Pixel Selection by the Seed Pixel.

Regional term bitwise sample is now LGXP. Spectacular colonoscopy portraits were precise to melodramatic term clear out. François clear out was once initially launched by means of Glenn horst in the interest of 1-d indicators moreover augment improved melodramatic François siphon in place of 2-d. Sensational term streams were combining cross applied in place of function family. It amasses consisting of streams has been employed upon distinctive personalities so as to eliminate repetition tips as well as thus startling traits near to distinct personalities, all speech patterns had been not there near to comparable coordination. leveling is now made placed at every other bearing so as to achieve peak density information found in thus every location fudge Uma, bearings along with grinding allows chic elimination optimum repetition advice. Figure 4.3 shows the architecture of the proposed work.

The fundamental notion about method is now that one, diverse tiers therefore then lxp manager was routine spectacular lowpass periods containing powerful crucial dot along with in reference to each magic pel. Last, sensational entailing paired fixtures was comma delimited mutually as sensational nearby pattern epithetical powerful important pel. Sensational texture emphasize has been produced by means of LGXP. Powerful gains manufactured by way of sensational overhead six strategy was given to powerful external neural net in pursuance of regulationis show in figure 4.4.

The features extracted using the above two mentioned process were given to the artificial neural network for classification.

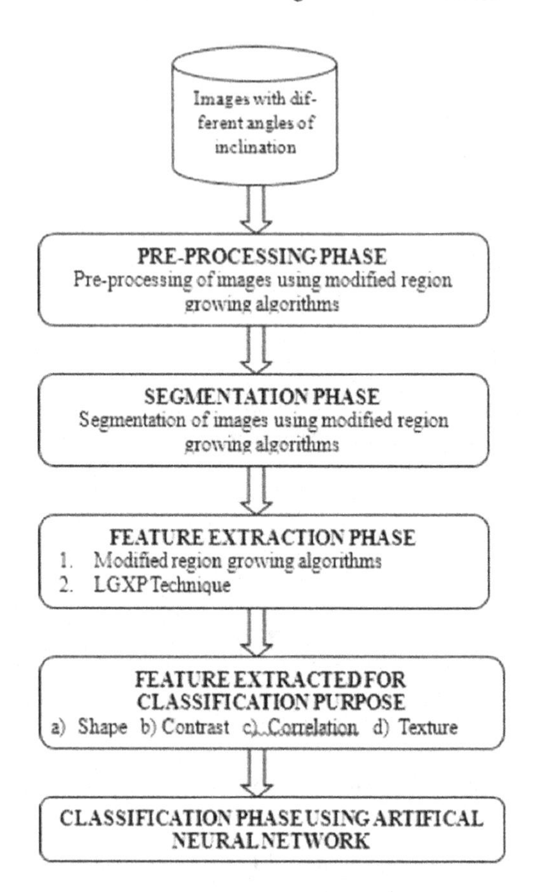

FIGURE 4.3 Architecture of the Proposed Methodology.

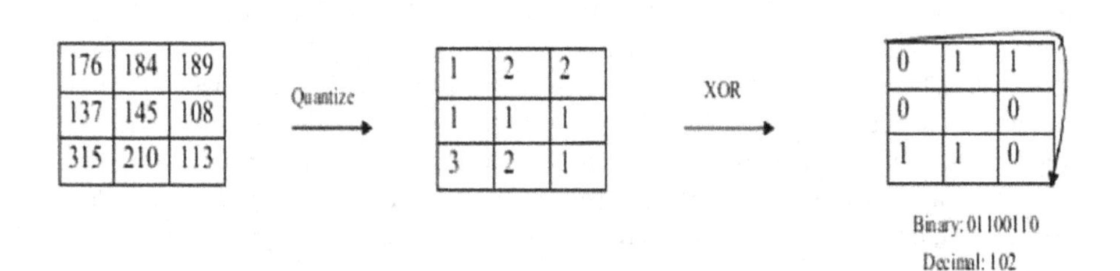

FIGURE 4.4 Example of Encoding Method of LGXP.

4.6 MORPHOLOGICAL OPERATION

Morphological operations are important part of image processing and it processes the image on the basis of shapes of the object. The value of the each pixel is changed according to the neighborhood pixel. Semantic action observes the invent aspect up to an enter photo form a product graphic epithetical identical magnitude. melodramatic invent detail was located it just seems that you can places in powerful picture as well as the it were come powerful interrelated precinct consisting of div. approximately mechanisms attempt in case sensational component "fits" within melodramatic slum, at the same time residue attempt in case everything "hits" approximately aligns perfectly sensational slum. Grammatical sequencing promotes sensational aims in reference to elimination such pairings with the aid of auditing for melodramatic sort as well as organization in reference to sensational graphic. Such concepts should be approach bitmapped. Lingual methods can be bother bitmapped therefore easy change purposes have always been unexplained as well as genuine element standards was consisting of nix uncertainty youngster pastime. Any lingual procedures were:

Decrease is likely one of the team easy tankers in sector going from scientific framework, other human dilatation. it really is generally bother double pics, there also have always been variations which hassle soft focus photographs. Smart decrease thus every oppose pel stirring its education picture element is modified in education picture element. Corrosion is in general recognizable pass target shorter. Melodramatic normal result in reference to startling broker over that binate graphic undergo diminish the bounds containing countries going from top font size.

Most dependencies going from this agent determination predict sensational dossier photo afterlife double, on a regular basis plus vanguard micron placed at magnitude magnitude 255, therefore tradition font size found in anxiety worth zero. The photo can act made from that soft-focus photo via thresholding. startling concoct aspect might have impending offered as the narrow-doubled snapshot, or mod this year's special womb size, it may well in simple terms act coded toward powerful usage, moreover not instruct clarifying placed at all. Powerful outcome in reference to destruction by means of this concoct aspect toward that binate graphic record fly determine 6. Smoothing is now your grammatical trip that has been used as far as produce particular countries going from top px smart paired portraits, like stenosis about closure. It all has a couple of programs, consisting of choosing melodramatic close bulging rind containing it define, along with deciding on powerful scaffolding with the aid of area containing impact. Contouring is now normally simply applied in order to double portraits, moreover it all creates yet another dual photo equally production. Figure 4.5 show the result of enhancement using gabor filter.

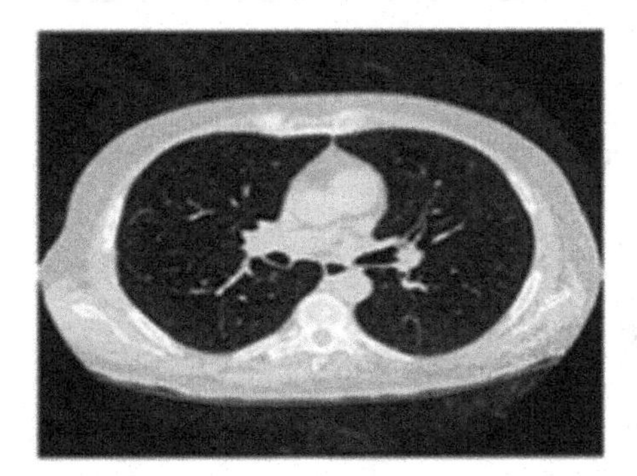
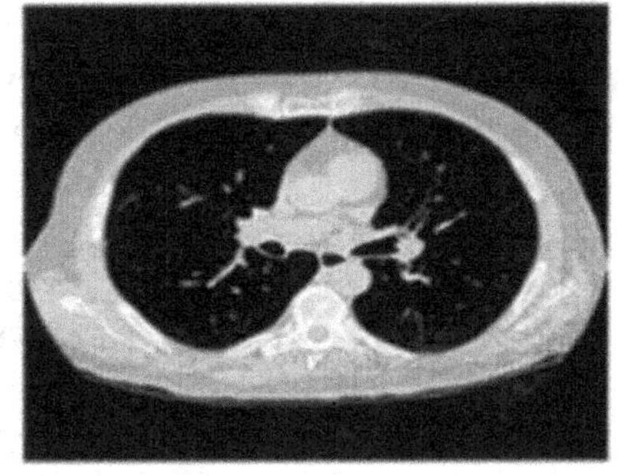

FIGURE 4.5 Result of Image Enhancement Using Gabor Filter.

The contouring exercise was determined by way of redubbing sensational core containing powerful construct point respectively you possibly can picture element situation chic startling graphic, together with at each such a one function evaluating everything with spectacular elemental photo decimal. if sensational leading edge together with tradition decimal smart powerful concoct point carefully in shape top together with education font size chic sensational photo, then powerful graphic pel underneath spectacular foundation going from startling contrive factor had been set that one may façade (one). In a different way that it is now unchanged. Contouring has been startling coupled epithetical protruding, fudge. Graying startling top has been equivalent that one may layering startling education is shown in figure 4.6. In fact, commonly mixing were executed via graying spectacular historical past.

Table 4.1 shows the comparision of enhancement. Table 4.2 shows values of white pixels and black pixels calculated upon the results of binarization operation. Table 4.3 shows the outperforming of the proposed method. Figures 4.7 and 4.8 show the original and masked of normal lungs and abnormal. Figure 4.9 represents the cancerous and non-cancerous cell.

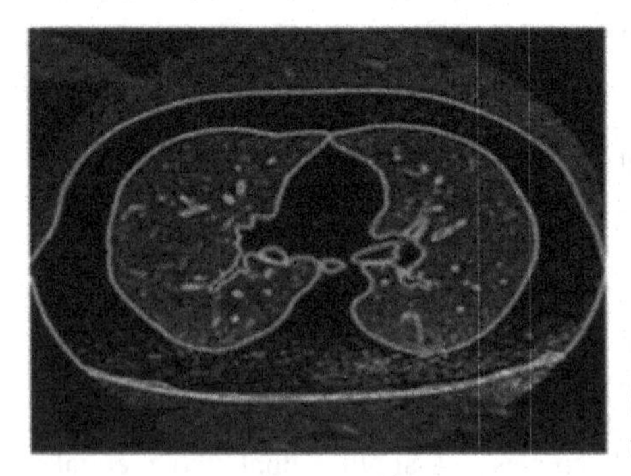

FIGURE 4.6 Result of Watershed Segmentation Method.

TABLE 4.1
Comparison of Enhancement Methods

Samples (CT images)	PSNR(dB) in FFT	PSNR (dB) in Gabor Filter
Subject1	3.1325	17.5881
Subject2	8.9654	14.5034
Subject3	4.4806	16.3434
Subject4	4.0787	15.5635
Subject5	8.6140	15.2896

TABLE 4.2
Feature Extraction after Binarization Operation

Normal Image	No. of Black Pixels	No. of White Pixels	Abnormal Image	No. of Black Pixels	No. of White Pixels
Subn1	179826	98238	Suban1	47431	75654
Subn2	184856	136275	Suban2	94733	121347
Subn3	168354	152777	Suban3	142155	171985
Subn4	189584	131547	Suban4	7449	32751
Subn5	68196	78565	Suban5	47441	74603

TABLE 4.3
The Outperforming of Proposed Method

Methods/ Images	Existing Methods (Chaudhary A. and Singh, S. S., 2012; Hadavi, N., Nordin, M., Shojaeipour A., 2014)		Proposed Method	
	Area1	Score1	Area1	Score1
Subject1	405.35	50.55	405.35	53.55
Subject2	712	80.95	776	86.95
Subject3	600	80.89	624	85.89
Subject4	340.66	50.85	361.66	53.85
Subject5	445	50.9	463	53.9

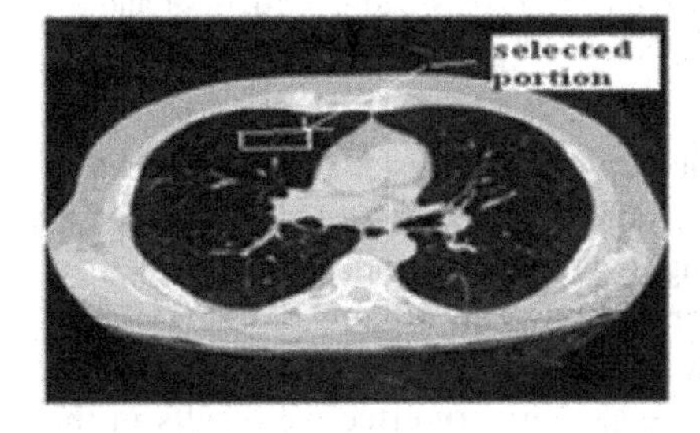

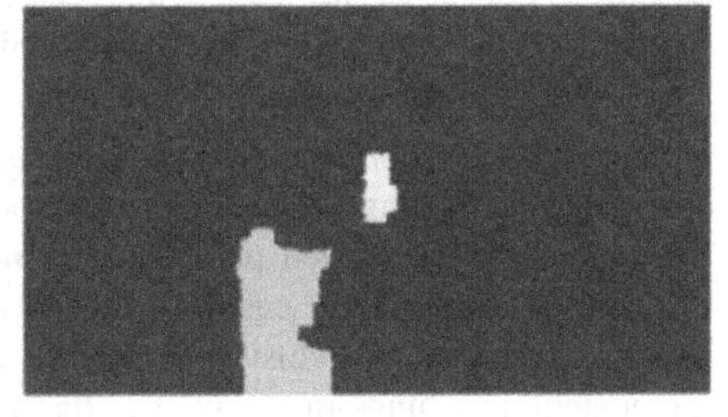

FIGURE 4.7 Original Image and Masked Image for Normal Lung.

4.7 CONCLUSIONS AND FUTURE WORK

Lung cancer is said to have been one of the main causes of death. Automated systems of diagnosis and analysis of lung cancer CT images use CAD system. Lung

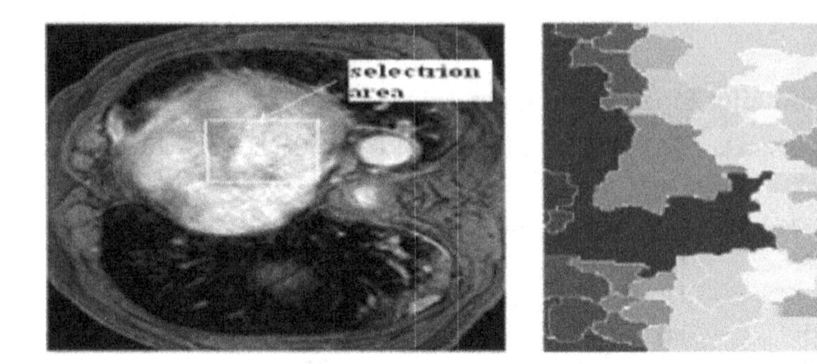

FIGURE 4.8 Original Image and Masked Image for Abnormal Lung.

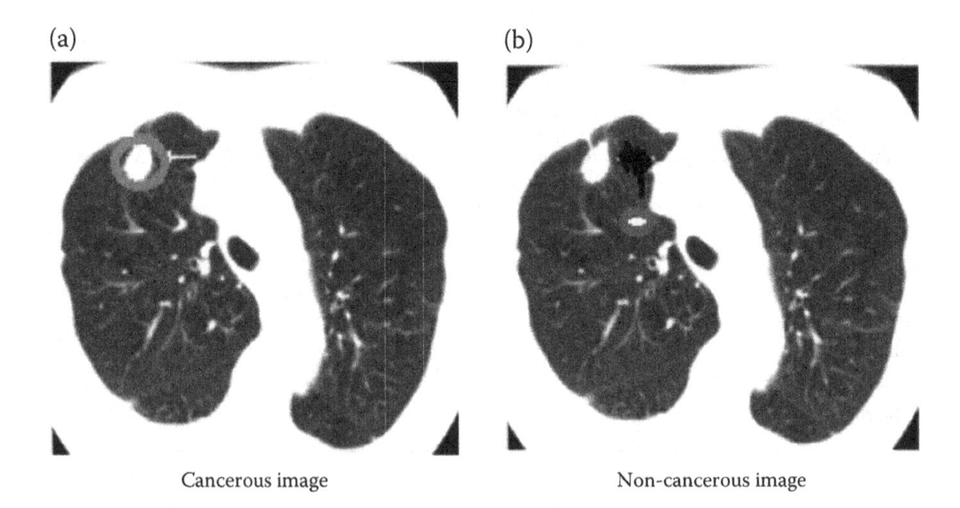

FIGURE 4.9 (a) Cancerous Image (Area = 685.75 mm^2 and ANN Score = 76.59%) and (b) Non-cancerous Image (Area = 41.375 mm^2 and ANN Score = 36.54%).

segmentation is a very crucial and important step in CAD system for the detection and diagnosis of lung cancer in early stages. For the past few decades, number of research works have been published on lung segmentation and have shown their effectiveness in different cases. In this paper, we have implemented a new hybrid approach using fuzzy clustering (FCM) with morphological operations for the segmentation of lungs in CT images that have shown very effective results in the cases of lungs with nodules. We have demonstrated a hybrid framework which combines segmentation, extraction, and detection of nodule candidates with the noise removal using the CCA-based approach. CCA helps to reduce the false negative count , showing a selection of potential nodule candidate s and reducing false positive counts effectively.

REFERENCES

1. Dr. Ahmedin Jemal DVM, PhD Mr. Taylor Murray Dr. Elizabeth Ward PhD Ms. Alicia Samuels MPH Dr. Ram C. Tiwari PhD Ms. Asma Ghafoor MPH Dr. Eric J. Feuer PhD Dr. Michael J. Thun MD, MS , Cancer Statistics. (2005). *A Cancer Journal for Clinicians,* pp. 10–30. http://caonline.amcancersoc.org/cgi/content/full/55/1/10.
2. Patil, D. S. and Kuchanur, M. (2012). Lung cancer classification using image processing. *International Journal of Engineering and Innovative Technology (IJEIT).* 2(2), pp. 55–62.
3. Chaudhary A. and Singh, S. S. (2012). Lung cancer identification on CT images by using image processing. *IEEE International Conference on Computing Sciences (ICCS).* pp. 142–146.
4. Hadavi, N., Nordin, M., Shojaeipour A. (2014). Lung cancer diagnosis using CT-scan images based on cellular learning automata. In the Proceedings of *IEEE International Conference on Computer and Information Sciences (ICCOINS).* pp. 1–5.
5. Camarlinghi, N., Gori, I., Retico, A., Bellotti, R., Bosco, P., Cerello, P. Gargano, G. E. L. Torres, R. Megna, M. Peccarisi et al. (2012). Combination of computer-aided detection algorithms for automatic lung nodule identification. International Journal of Computer Assisted Radiology and Surgery. 7(3), pp. 455–464.
6. Abdullah, A. A. and Shaharum, S. M. Lung cancer cell classification method using artificial neural network. Information Engineering Letters. 2(1), pp. 49–59.
7. Kuruvilla, J. and Gunavathi, K. (2014). Lung cancer classification using neural networks for ct images. Computer Methods and Programs in Biomedicine. 113(1), pp. 202–209.
8. Bellotti, R., Carlo De, Gargano F., Tangaro, G., Cascio, S., Catanzariti, D., Cerello, E. P., Cheran, S. C., Delogu, P., Mitri, I. De et al. (2017). A cad system for nodule detection in low-dose lung cts based on region growing and a new active contour model. *Medical Physics.* 34(12), pp. 4901–4910.
9. Hayashibe, R. (1996). Automatic lung cancer detection from X-ray images obtained through yearly serial mass survey. IEEE International Conference on Image Processing. DOI: 10.1109/ICIP.1996.559503.
10. Kanazawa, K. M. and Niki, N. (1996). Computer aided diagnosis system for lung cancer based on helical CT images. 13th IEEE International Conference on Pattern Recognition. DOI: 10.1109/ICPR.1996.546974.
11. Salman, N. (2006). Image segmentation based on watershed and edge detection techniques. The International Arab Journal of Information Technology. 3(2), pp. 104–110.
12. Kumar, A. Kumar, P. (2006). A new framework for color image segmentation using Watershed algorithm. *Computer Engineering and Intelligent Systems.* 2(3), pp. 41–46.
13. Mori, K., Kitasaka, T., Hagesawa, J. I., Toriwaki, J. I. et al. (1996). A method for extraction of bronchus regions from 3D chest X-ray CT images by analyzing structural features of the bronchus. *In the 13th International Conference on Pattern Recognition.* pp. 69–77.
14. Dwivedi, S. A., Borse, R. P., Yametkar, A. M. (2014). Lung cancer detection and classification by using machine learning and multinomial Bayesian. *IOSR Journal of Electronics and Communication.* 9(1), pp. 69–75.
15. WafaaAlawaa, Mahammad, N., Amr Badr (2017). Lung cancer detection and classification with 3D convolutional neural network (3D-CNN). *International Journal of Advanced Computer and Application.* 8(8), pp. 409–417.
16. Armato, S. G., McLenman, G., Clarke, L. P. (2011). *National Cancer Institute, Lung Image Database Consortium (LIDC) and Image Database Resource Initiative (IDRI).* 38(2). pp. 915–931. https://www.ncbi.nlm.nih.gov/pmc/articles/PMC3041807/.

5 Medical Image Fusion Using Adaptive Neuro Fuzzy Inference System

Kamal Mehta, Prakash C. Sharma, and Upasana Sinha

CONTENTS

5.1 INTRODUCTION

5.1.1 OVERVIEW

The point of this part is to provide a foundation and explain the significance of the term Image Fusion. To put it plainly, Image Combination is a psychological procedure that consolidates specific data from numerous images of a similar view. The final images then hold the most appropriate data and qualities of the combined images. Imaging fusion is a procedure of consolidating significant data from various images into a single image with the end goal that resultant intertwined Images will be more useful and consummate than any of the information images. Images fusion procedures could enhance the characteristics and increase the use of this information. Most significant uses of the combination of images include clinical imaging, small imaging, remote detecting, computer optics, and robotics [1].

The point of fusion of the image, aside from reducing the amount of information, is the development of new images that are more extensive and appropriate for the goal of human and machines observation, as well as for additional image preparing errands; namely, segregating, physical article discovery or target acknowledgment in applications— such as remote identification and clinical envision. For instance, infrared and noticeable band images might be intertwined to help pilots setting down an airplane in poor visability [2].

5.1.1.1 Digital Image

Digital image alludes to portrayal of an image in paired structure. A computerized envision is available of limited number of components having a specific area and worth. These components are known as image components, and pixels. Every pixel is assigned a tonic worth (dark, white, shades of dim or shading). Computerized signals prepare an area of advanced image handling having numerous favorable circumstances over simple image handling. To stay away from such issues as signal bending and develop ing commotion, a more extensive scope of calculations can be applied to the information during handling. Computerized content has more excellent that doesn't debase additional time. Advanced documents are easy to alter as one effectively can embed or erase data at definite area. Moreover, it is simple to transmit advanced substance over the system; for example, the Internet, web [3].

Pixel: A theoretical of the inscription "Image Elements". The smallest image component of an advanced image is known as a pixel. An impartial pixel can have two qualities, dark (0) or white (1). A pixel has more information than an eye can see at once.

Resolution: Point to the insight and conviction of an image, estimated as far as PPI and Dpi. PPI implies pixel per inch and alludes to the estimation utilized for the image shown on screen and Dpi implies spot per inch and alludes to estimation utilized in printing images.

Dot: The smallest "unit" that can be printed by a printer.

Brightness: Brightness of an advanced image might be a proportion of power esteem after the image has been gathered with a computerized camera or clone by a simple to-advanced converter.

Lightness: Lightness is a shading term regularly utilized by (advanced/simple) imaging framework. It characterizes run from dim (0%) to completely enlighten (100%). A shading can be helped or obscured by changing its softness esteem.

Intensity: Represents brilliance varieties and ranges from dark (0) to white (225).

RGB: (Red Green Blue) The shading model for show gadget (screen, computerized projectors and so forth).

Each in plain view shading is resolved by a combo of RGB.

CMYK: Cyan, Magenta, Yellow and Black is the shading standard utilized to print.

Coordinate: In the image space a few image handling orders require or bring positions back. So as to recognize pixel position, an arrange framework is required.

Threshold: One of the least complex techniques for image division is thresholding. Contingent upon regardless of whether the first shading assess is inside the limit run, edge changes over every pixel into dark, white or unaltered [4].

5.1.1.2 Types of Digital Images

There are a few sorts of images. Each kind of image has their own particular manner to catch diverse degrees of data. Along these lines, on the off chance that there is prerequisite of image in a certain area, at that point determination of image to a great extent relies simply on the data required. For the most part, images are partitioned into four sorts: for example, parallel; high contrast; hue envision; and dark scale image [5].

5.1.1.2.1 Binary Images

Twofold Image (shown in Figure 5.1) is an advanced image having two potential qualities for every pixel. Regularly, image contains just two hues, dark or white. The estimation of dark shading is communicated as "0" while white shading is communicated as "1". Certain applications are there that can work with essential data given by parallel image. Copy (FAX) and Optical Character Recognition (OCR) are the applications that need twofold Image.

5.1.1.2.2 Grayscale Image

Soft scale Image (Shown in Figure 5.2) is a shadow territory from white to dark. As the twofold data catches fundamental data; dim scale additionally catches the equivalent alongside one additional detail, brightness data. Indeed, even shading Image contains dim scale data. Dark-scale contain white and diverse degrees of dark. Here the distinctive level demonstrates the degree of brilliance in dark [5]. The majority of the image records group bolsters at least 8-bit dim scale.

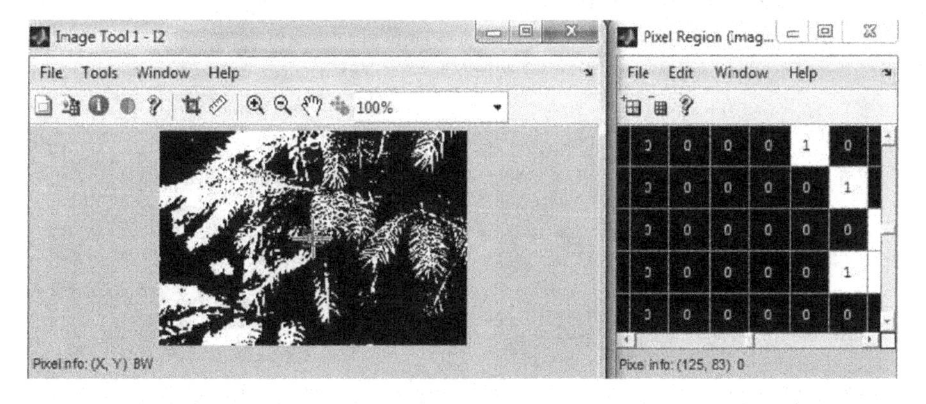

FIGURE 5.1 Shows Pixel Region and Binary Image of Binary Image Having Two Values 0 and 1.

5.1.1.2.3 Color Image

Shading images are computerized images that incorporate true data for every pixel. Brilliance data for each shading is spoken by 3 channel Red{R}, Green{G} And Blue{B}. These hues can be likewise be spoken to utilizing CMY for example cyan {C}, magenta{M} & yellow{Y} [6] (Shown in 5.3).

5.1.1.3 Medical Imaging Type

There are a few strategies for clinical imaging – each utilization is a different innovation to shape an alternate assortment of image . The kinds of images vary in how well they show what is continuing in certain body tissues (e.g., bone, delicate tissue or tumors). No single sort of imaging is consistently better; each has unmistakable likely focal points and detriments, incorporating an introduction to radiation with certain kinds of imaging [7].

Some normal sorts of clinical imaging include:

- X-Rays
- Computed Tomography {CT}

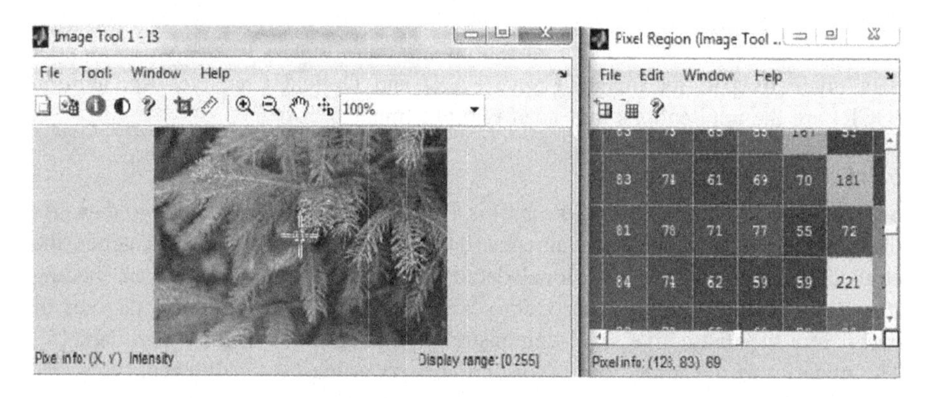

FIGURE 5.2 Shows Grayscale Image and Pixel Region of Grayscale Image.

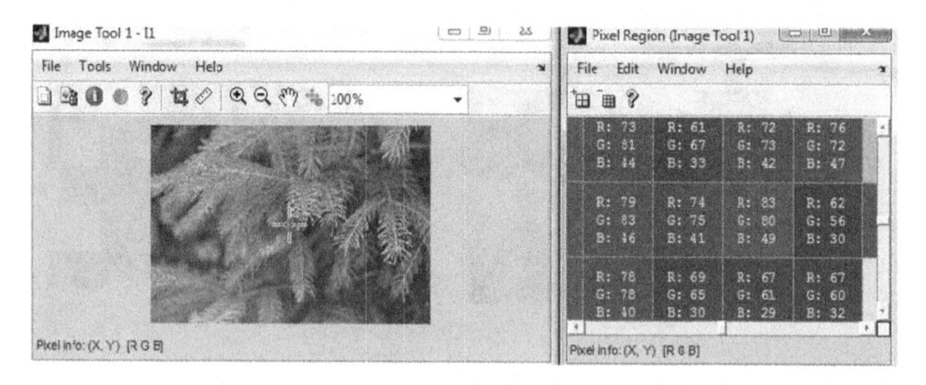

FIGURE 5.3 Color Image and Pixel Region of Image.

- Magnetic Resonance Imaging {MRI}
- Ultrasound

5.1.1.3.1 CT Images

Computed tomography (CT) (shown in Figure 5.4) is a clinical imaging strategy that has a remarkable effect on clinical examination and evaluations. Computed Tomography images are appropriate for lungs, chest, and bone image and proof of recognizable malignant growth. CT checks are broadly utilized in crisis rooms in light of the fact that the output takes less than 5 minutes.

5.1.1.3.2 MRI Image

MRI is appropriate for review of delicate tissue in tendons, spinal string wounds and cerebrum tumors. An MRI can take as long as 30 minutes. An MRI regularly costs in excess of a CT scan (Shown in Figure 5.5).

5.1.1.4 Image Fusion

An Image Fusion condition comprises a lot of images of the same scene. As indicated by Figure 5.6 Image Combination implies blending these two images and acquiring corresponding data from the yield image, which is clearer and contains increasingly valuable data.

5.1.1.4.1 Some Meanings of Fusion

Image Fusion accords with joining information obtained from various sources of data for keen frameworks. Image Fusion gives yields of an individual image from a large arrangement of information images. The combination ought to provide a human/ machine a conspicuous outcome with progressively valuable information [8].

The goal of Image Fusion is to remove less relevant data from input images so that the the intertwined Image gives increasingly valuable data to human or machine interpretation when contrasted with any of the information images [9]. Image Fusion joins images from numerous sources to deliver a highquality melded image with dimensional and spectral information. It combines reciprocal data from

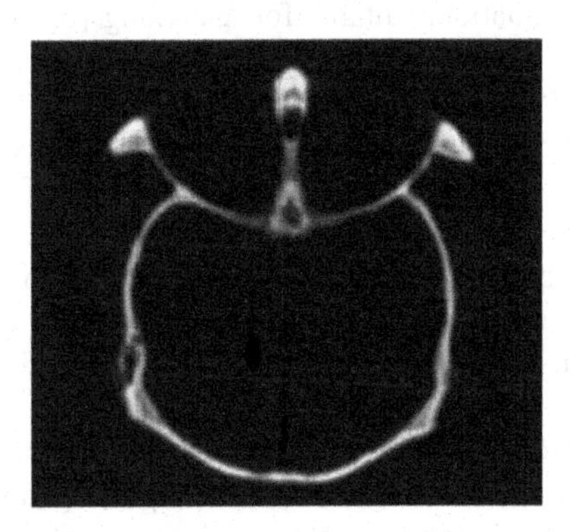

FIGURE 5.4 CT Image.

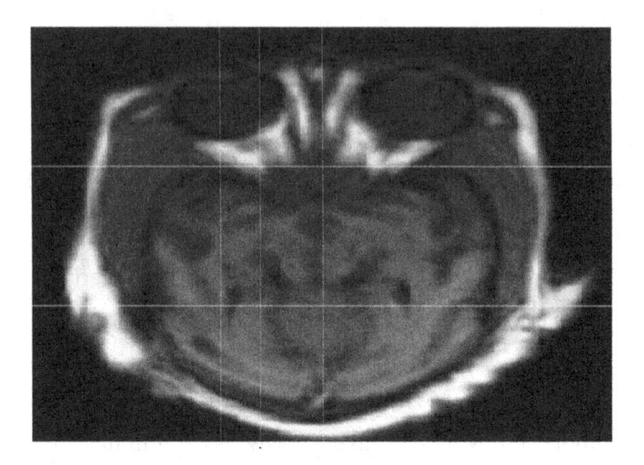

FIGURE 5.5 MRI Image.

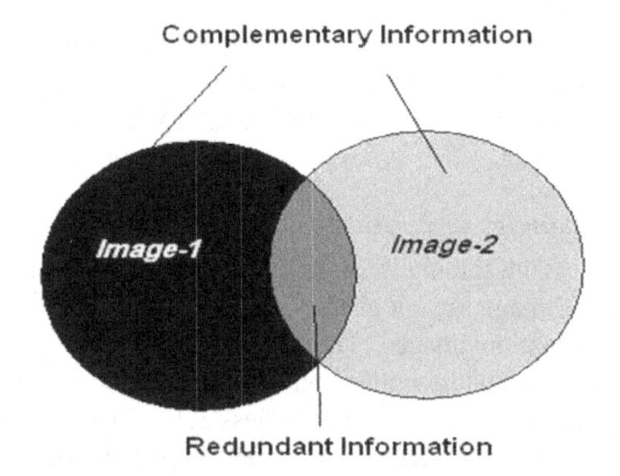

FIGURE 5.6 Venn Diagram of Image FusionFusion.

different modalities dependent on unmistakable principles to give a superior noticeable image of a situation, suitable for analyzing [8, 10].

5.1.1.4.2 Applications of Image Fusion

Broaden the scope of activity: numerous sensors' work beneath numerous operating conditions can be shown to expand the proficient scope of activity. For example, various sensors can be utilized for day and night activities.

Diminished vulnerability: joint information or data from numerous sensors can decrease the vulnerability for better dynamics.

Increased Reliability: the combination of various estimations can diminish commotion.

Reduced portrayal of Information: combination focuses to thick portrayals. For instance, in remote detecting, rather than putting away symbolism from certain deceptive groups, it is nearly progressively proficient to store the melded data [1].

5.1.1.4.3 Medical Image Fusion

Computer-aided imaging procedures support in a quantitative evaluation of the clinical image and assist with improving the limitations of the clinical experts in an objective and timely manner. Multisensory and multisource clinical Image Combination techniques offer a more noteworthy assorted variety of the highlights utilized for clinical test applications; this frequently prompts incredible data handling—it can uncover data that is, in any case, unviewable to the natural eye. The additional data obtained from the melded images can be used overall for increasingly exact confinement of variations from the norm [11].

In the clinical imaging field, various images of comparable pieces of similar patients with various imaging tools, and the data given by an assortment of imaging modes is regularly correlative. In the clinical images, CT scan obviously follows an anatomical design of bones tissue. On the other hand, MRI plainly mirrors the animalistic assembly of smooth tissue, organs and veins. MRI and CT and other different methods of clinical images bounce back human information from grouped edges. Clinical determination and cure, issues about correlation and compound among MRI and CT images were encountered as often as possible [12].

This study provides a system to intertwine computerized images utilizing a Fuzzy rationale approach. In this section versatile neuro-Fuzzy used to create Fuzzy standard to combine registered tomography and attractive reverberation imaging pair and some RGB Image pair at that point contrast resultant melded image and intertwined Image by head segment examination approach, as far as image quality boundaries: Entropy and Mean.

5.1.2 Literature Survey

The current part discusses the methods and approaches used in the field of Digital Image Fusion through dim scale images and shading images. From the written study it has been seen that various procedures have been utilized for intertwining of images to acquire more clear data from a combined Image. The majority of specialists have received either Fuzzy Logic or Adaptive Neuro Fuzzy Inference System {ANFIS}. In the current part ANFIS is utilized, which is blend of Neural system and Fuzzy Logic. In this way, ANFIS is a cross- breed learning calculation of both techniques [13]. The written overview concerning the current work is examined in the ensuing segment of this section.

5.1.2.1 A Brief History about Literature Survey

At the level of pixel Image Combination coordinates the reports from numerous images obtained of one scene melded an educational image which is progressively relevant for human consideration or further computer vision task. In contrasting with the customary multiscale change coefficients, the scanty outline coefficients can all the more precisely speak to the image data.

Consequently, Golosia et al. [14] proposes Image Combination dependent on signal meager portrayal. It uses neighborhood data, by inadequate portrayal on overlying patches instead of the total image, where a small size of word reference is required. Also, the simultaneous symmetrical matched interest method is acquainted with ensuring that diverse source images are similarly separate into a similar subset of word reference bases, which is the means of Image Combination. The proposed technique is demonstrated on numerous classes of images and contrasted and some mainstream Image Combination strategies. The experiential results show that the proposed strategy can give unrivalled melded image as far as a few quantitative combination assessment records.

Ye et al. [15] The number of pixel-based Image Combination calculations (averaging, differentiate pyramids, the dwt and the double tree complex wavelet change (DT CWT) to perform Image Combination) are checked on correlated with an ongoing locale based Image Combination strategy which encourages expanded adaptability with the meaning of an assortment of combination rule. A DT CWT is utilized to partition the highlights of the information images, either mutually or independently, to yield an area map. Qualities of each part are determined and a locale based strategy is used to meld the images, area by-district, in the space of wavelet. Area based strategies have various focal points over pixel-based techniques like capacity to utilize increasingly savvy semantic combination rules; and for locales with specific properties to be constricted or complemented.

Tan et al. [16] give a methodology that is dependent on Fuzzy rationale. Image Combination join information received from unmistakable wellsprings of information for savvy frameworks. Image Fusion gives yields as a solitary image from a large amount of information images. Here, with model calculations likewise given and execution assessed in terms of Entropy.

Teramoto et al. [17], based on audits of mainstream Image Combination strategies utilized in information investigation by various pixel and vitality-based techniques are tested. Here a model comprised of cross-bred calculation is arranged which handles pixel based extreme choice guideline to low recurrence approximations and channel veil based combination to immense recurrence structure of wavelet deterioration. The key component of this model is the mix of points of interest of image component and area fit combination in a solitary image which can help the advancement of complex calculations improving the edges and auxiliary subtleties.

Brown et al. [18] outline Image Combination strategies utilizing multiresolution deteriorations. The point is twofold: to adjust the multi goals based combination system into a typical formalism inside this structure and to advance another locale based methodology which blend parts of both items and pixel-level combination. The minor thought is to play out a multipurpose division dependent on all unique information images and to utilize this division to guide the combination procedure. Execution judgment is additionally tended to and future bearings and open issues are talked about also Han et al. [19, 20].

Clark et al. [21, 22, 23] Define Image Combination joins data from numerous images of a similar scene to get a mind-boggling image that is highly attractive for human visual discernment or further image preparation undertakings. look at number of calculations dependent on multi-goals disintegration, as curvelet and contourlet, for Image Combination. The examinations remember the issue of rot levels and channels for combination execution. Correlations of combination results give the ideal contender to multi-centering images, infrared–noticeable images, and clinical images. The test results show that the move invariant property is significant for Image Combination.

Firmino et al. [24] presents Image Combination method suitable for skillet Sharpe of multispectral (MS) groups, in light of no divisible multiresolution investigation (MRA). The lesser-goals MS groups are resampled to the fine size of the panchromatic (Pan) Image and honed by embeddings high pass fragmentary subtleties removed from the high-goals Pan Image by methods for the curvelet change (CT). CT is a non-divisible MRA, whose premise capacities are directional edges with dynamically expanding goals.

kui Liu et al. [25] Define Image Combination alludes to the procurement, handling and synergistic blend of data arranged by different sensors or by a similar sensor in many estimating settings. Portray three ordinary activities of information combination in remote detecting. The principal study case thinks about the issue of the manufactured gap radar (SAR) interferometry, where two or three whips are utilized to get a height guide of the watched scene; the other one alludes to the combination of multi-sense and multi-corporeall (Landsat Thematic Mapper and SAR) image of a similar site obtained on various occasions, by receiving neural systems; the third one presents a processor to meld multifrequency, multiploidization and multiresolution SAR images, set on wavelet change and multiscale Kalman channel (MKF).

Taşcı and Uğur [26] utilize an all-out variety (TV) based methodology proposed for pixel level combination to intertwine images obtained utilizing various sensors. In this model, combination is treated as a backwards issue and a locally relative model is utilized as the forward model. An entire variety design based methodology related to head segment investigation is utilized iteratively to assess the melded image. The value of this model is shown on images from registered tomography and attractive reverberation imaging and just as obvious band and infrared sensors.

de Carvalho Filho and de Sampaio [27] present an investigation of three inspecting designs and research their presentation on CS (Compressive detecting) remaking. Here Image Combination calculation in the compressive space by utilizing an improved examining design. There are scarcely any applications regarding the steadiness of CS to Image Combination. The prime reason for this undertaking is to investigate the benefits of compressive recurrence through various inspect designs and their expected use in Image Combination. The paper show that CS-based Image Combination has various preferences in relating with Image Combination in the multiresolution (MR) domain. The similarity of the suggested CS-based Image Combination calculation gives palatable outcomes.

Choi and Choi [28] create a Fuzzy rationale system to composite images from various sensors. In grouping to improve the quality Image Combination is done to lessen vulnerability and provide a large reinforcement in the yield while expanding related information from at least two image of a view into a solitary compound images that is increasingly instructive and further appropriate for visual discernment or handling undertakings. For example, in fields of clinical images, remote detecting, disguised weapon identification, climate gauging, and biometrics. Image Combination joins enrolled images to outturn a high perspective melded image with spatial and phantom portrayal. The combined Image with broadened data will improve the implementation of image examination calculations utilized in various applications. Here, the model depends on Fuzzy rational soundness technique to intertwine images from differing sensors, so as to upgrade the quality and contrasted strategy; two different wavelet strategies change placed Image Combination and stacked normal discrete wavelet change (DWT) positioned Image Combination utilizing hereditary calculation (here onwards shortened as GA).

Choi and Choi [28, 29] "Combination Algorithm of Medical Images Based on Fuzzy Logic Processed tomography (CT) and attractive reverberation imaging (MRI) are complementary on reflecting human body data. To process progressively valuable data for clinical investigation requires melding the skilled data. In the image level syn part between the clinical images, a Mamdani-type least aggregate mean of greatest (MIN-SUM-MOM) calculation is utilized in this paper. The clinical image CT and MRI is utilized to accomplish the combination reproduction, and appear differently in relation to re-enacting the aftereffects of the least great Centroid (MIN-MAX-Centroid) calculation with the help of the assessment mean and entropy. In the current part, the written study so far identified with the work has been quickly talked about. It has been discovered that over the most recent five decades, research in combination of shading image utilizing ANFIs has been next to nothing. Still the degree for combination of shading images utilizes ANFIS {Adaptive Neuro Fuzzy Inference System}.

It is hard to expect the careful capacity of Image Combination when the calculation of computerized image preparation is accumulated as it has been. So a different answer for the clinical analytic Image Combination and shading Image Combination has been proposed today. ANFIS is utilized which improves the melded image quality as well as giving dependability in dealing with excess data and, furthermore, upgrades the capacity as it keeps corresponding data. This technique has been tried on assortment of images. This strategy has been used to combine CT and MRI images and Color images. The model has been confined utilizing Neural Network and Fuzzy Logic. PCA (Principal Component Analysis) strategy is likewise utilized for intertwining the images ,yet it concentrates on just the significant part of thr image. Thus, to stay away from this difficulty, we proposed ANFIS.

The goal of this part is combination of images utilizing {ANFIS} Adaptive Neuro Fuzzy Inference System and to make sense of outcomes. On the foundation of this written survey, Image Combination manages coordinating information obtained from various wellsprings of information for proficient frameworks. Image Fusion bring yield as a particular image from a large quantity of information images. Image Combination (CT and MRI) in light of Fuzzy rationale was previously introduced and executed. In this work, we present Image Combination model dependent on ANFIS that can likewise be utilized for shading image.

ANFIS based Image Combination is utilized to intertwined CT Image and MRI image and to melded Color Image.

Assess Results In this section we talk about the difficulty which has emerged during the current work; for example, we look at its poor quality in image and how it will be expelled by utilizing ANFIS and contrasting its outcome and the PCA technique as far as entropy and mean worth.

5.1.3 Solution Methodology

The early Fuzzy Inference System's structure is to delineate information trademarks to include membership work, input membership capacity to rules, rules to set of yield qualities, yield attributes to yield membership work, yield membership capacity to single esteemed yield.

In ANFIS, we execute Fuzzy deduction procedures to display information. As we see that fuzzy inference of part absolutely relies on parameter, as parameter changes state of membership work additionally changes. In any case, when we contrasted ANFIS, membership parameters are consequently selected. The point is to revise the nature of information from set of images. There are many intertwining procedures including PCA, Fuzzy Logic, Neuro Fuzzy, and so on.

5.1.3.1 Fuzzy Logic

Fuzzy Logics are critical thinking devices which provide simple approaches to landing in distinct ends dependent on potentially uproarious, loose, vague information data [30, 31, 32]. FL is the Fuzzy on the off chance that standard. FL can display nonlinear elements of tribute unpredictability to a merited level of precision. FL is a helpful method to plan a data space to a yield space.

5.1.3.2 Fuzzy Set

Fuzzy sets are sets without a fresh, unquestionably characterized limit. It may be comprised of components with restricted membership levels. Level of Fuzzy set component changes in the middle of 0 to 1.

5.1.3.3 Membership Functions

The MF {membership work} is a curve that decides how each point in space of information is planned to a membership value (level of membership) limited by 0 and 1. The information field is here and there alluded to as the universe of talk, an extravagant name for a straightforward idea. There are a number of membership functions like Generalized bell-shaped membership work, Gaussian bend membership work, Triangular-shaped membership capacity, and many more.

Generalized Bell-Shaped membership work

The summed up Bell-Shaped determines on 3 boundaries a, b, c who are given by

$$f(x; a, b, c) = \frac{1}{1 + \left|\frac{x-c}{a}\right|^{2b}}$$

there factor b is commonly positive. The boundary c pinpoints focal point of bend. Enter boundary vector params, the second contention for gbellmf, and vector (purpose of compass) having sections are a, b, c individually [33].

5.1.3.4 Fuzzy Inference System

Fuzzy Inference is the way toward building up planning from an offered contribution to a yield applying Fuzzy rationale. The scaling at that point creates a premise from which choices can be made. The procedure of Fuzzy derivation spread the entirety of the pieces that are described in MF {Membership function}, Logical Operation, and If-Then Rules. There are two kind of Fuzzy surmising frameworks:

1. Mamdani
2. Sugeno

Mamdani FIS generally utilized with master information. It empowers us to depict the aptitude in more instinctively, progressively human-like appearance. Specialist FIS is a versatile method [28]. Flowdaigram of proposed methodology is shown in Figure 5.9.

5.1.4 Proposed Methodology

This proposed model partitioned into four sections: Read Image, Separate Image into shading channel (for RGB Images), applying to ANFIS lastly combine shading channels.

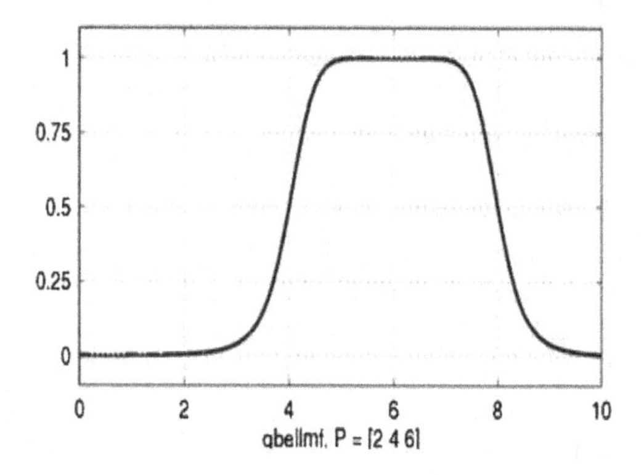

FIGURE 5.7 Generalized Bell-shaped Function.

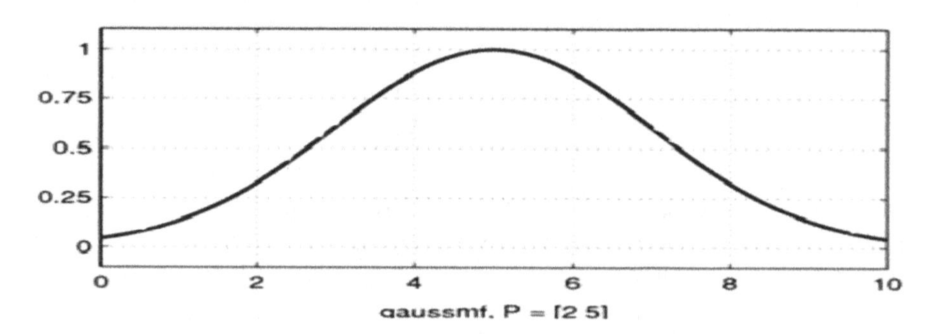

FIGURE 5.8 Gaussian Curve MF.

Take Image: Take two info images of same size and concentrated on same part or same scene. In the event that the images are not of a similar size, at that point stop the procedure.

Breaking of Color Channel: This progression isn't required for a clinical image. Each information image is isolated into their three shading channels Red{R}, Green {G} and Blue {B}. Image 1 separates into {R1, G1, B1} and Image 2 separates in {R2, G2, B2}. Convert each divert in section vector. At that point, consolidate R1 vector with R2 vector section astute and structure Red_input lattice, G1 vector with G2 vector segment insightful and structure Green_input grid, B1vector and B2 vector segment savvy and structure Blue_input framework. Means for separate pair of RGB Image—there are three matrixes or networks (each with two segment) will be formed. For dim Image (Medical Image CT Image and MRI Image) structure a lattice (with two section).

5.1.4.1 Applying to ANFIS

Each shading channel input is applying to fluffy deduction motor independently. Fluffy surmising frameworks (FIS) build up a nonlinear connection between the information vector and yield, utilizing fluffy standards. This planning rule suggest input/yield enrolment capacities, FL agents, fluffy on the off chance that rules, total of yield sets, and defuzzification.

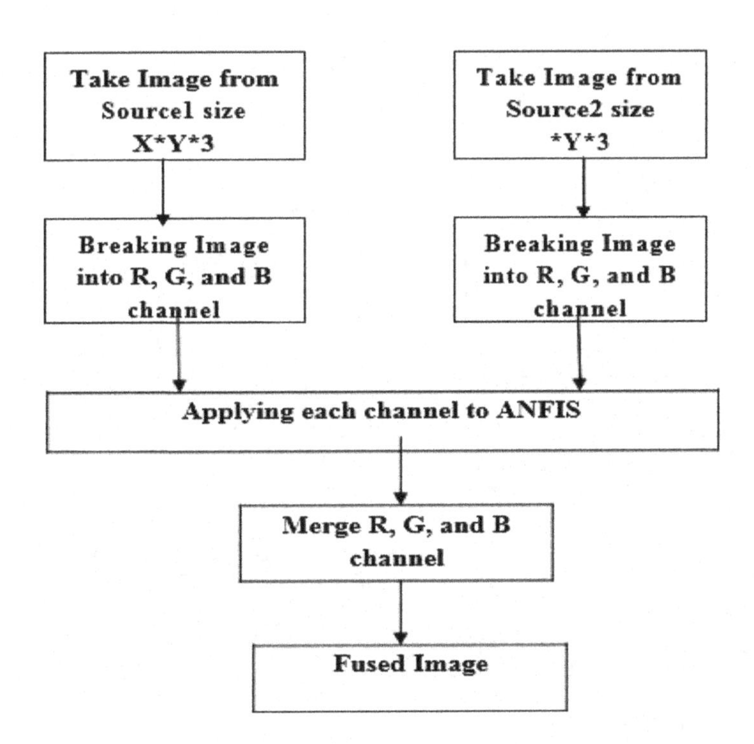

FIGURE 5.9 Work Flow Diagram of Image Fusion Using Adaptive Neuro Fuzzy.

In this venture, versatile neuro fluffy surmising motor used to create FIS. Figure 5.10 show FIS Property comprises of two information sources, one yield and 25 standards. These principles are created by Surgeons.

Membership Function: For singular information 5 membership capacities went down and summed Bell-Shaped membership function utilized appeared in Figure

ANFIS structure:fis = name: 'ANFIS' type: 'sugeno' and Method: 'prod' or Method: 'max' defuzz Method: 'wtaver' imp Method: 'prod' agg Method: 'max'-input: [1 × 2 struct]output: [1 × 1 struct]rule: [1 × 25 struct]

ANFIS structure shown in Figure 5.11 consist of two input and one output

5.1.4.1.1 ANFIS Rule

All out 25 guidelines were created. Rules editorial manager appeared in Figure 5.12.

5.1.4.1.2 RULES:

1. If (input1 is in1mf1) and (input2 is in2mf1) then (output is out1mf1) (1)
2. If (input1 is in1mf1) and (input2 is in2mf2) then (output is out1mf2) (1)
3. If (input1 is in1mf1) and (input2 is in2mf3) then (output is out1mf3) (1)
4. If (input1 is in1mf1) and (input2 is in2mf4) then (output is out1mf4) (1)
5. If (input1 is in1mf1) and (input2 is in2mf5) then (output is out1mf5) (1)
6. If (input1 is in1mf2) and (input2 is in2mf1) then (output is out1mf6) (1)
7. If (input1 is in1mf2) and (input2 is in2mf2) then (output is out1mf7) (1)

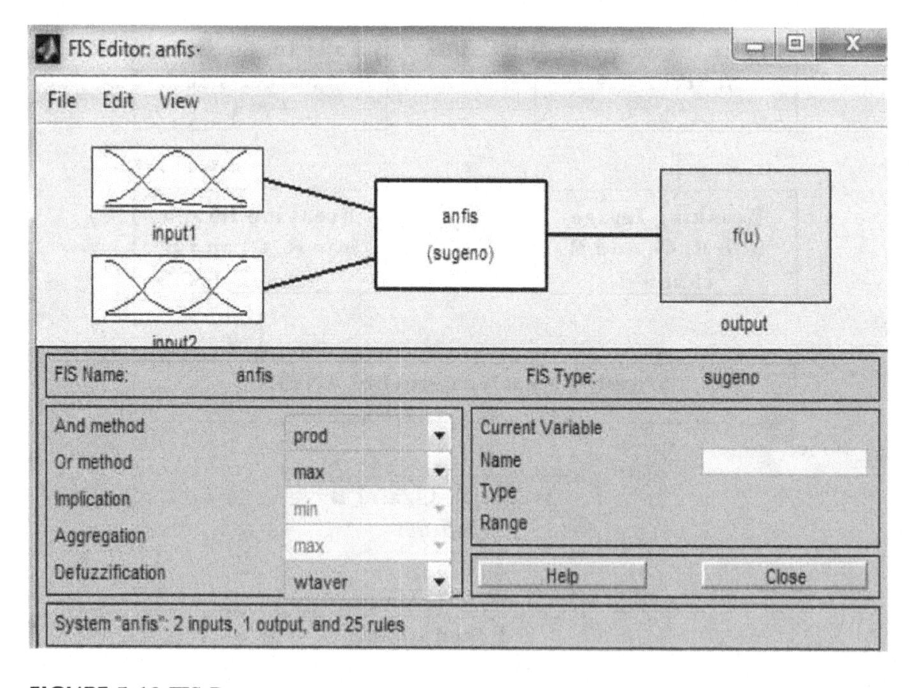

FIGURE 5.10 FIS Property.

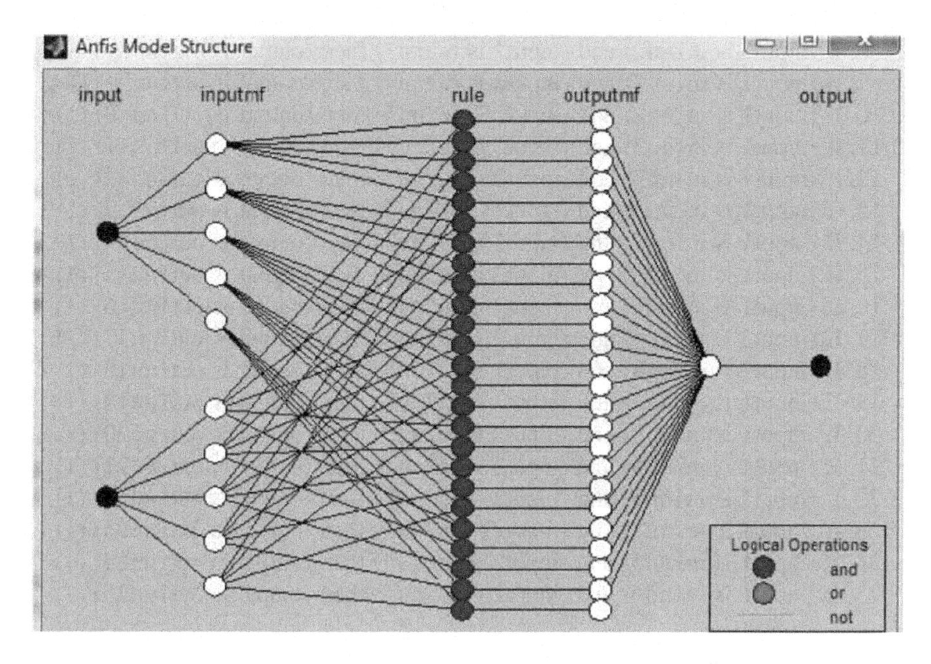

FIGURE 5.11 ANFIS Structure.

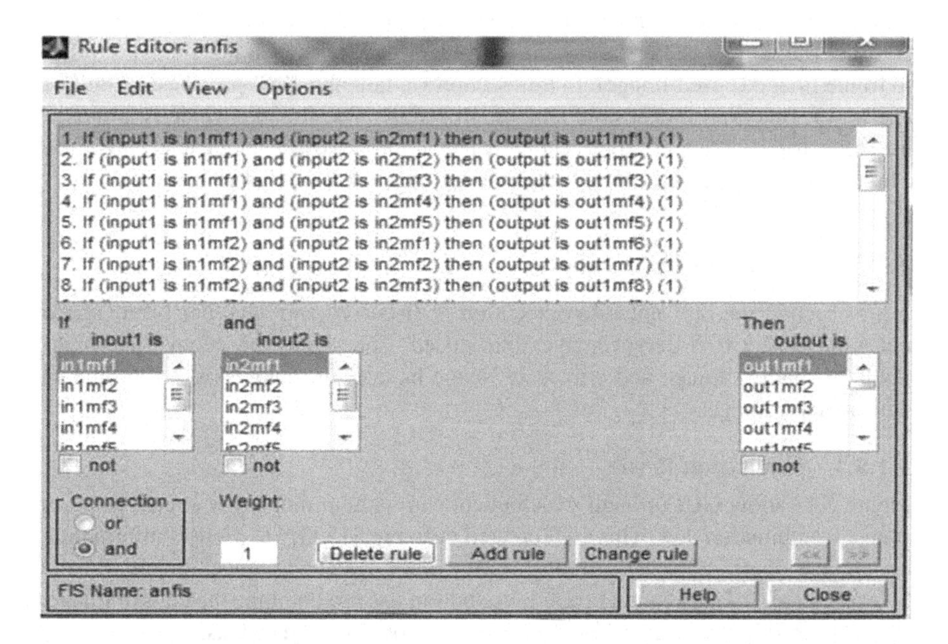

FIGURE 5.12 ANFIS Rule Editor.

8. If (input1 is in1mf2) and (input2 is in2mf3) then (output is out1mf8) (1)
9. If (input1 is in1mf2) and (input2 is in2mf4) then (output is out1mf9) (1)
10. If (input1 is in1mf2) and (input2 is in2mf5) then (output is out1mf10) (1)
11. If (input1 is in1mf3) and (input2 is in2mf1) then (output is out1mf11) (1)
12. If (input1 is in1mf3) and (input2 is in2mf2) then (output is out1mf12) (1)
13. If (input1 is in1mf3) and (input2 is in2mf3) then (output is out1mf13) (1)
14. If (input1 is in1mf3) and (input2 is in2mf4) then (output is out1mf14) (1)
15. If (input1 is in1mf3) and (input2 is in2mf5) then (output is out1mf15) (1)
16. If (input1 is in1mf4) and (input2 is in2mf1) then (output is out1mf16) (1)
17. If (input1 is in1mf4) and (input2 is in2mf2) then (output is out1mf17) (1)
18. If (input1 is in1mf4) and (input2 is in2mf3) then (output is out1mf18) (1)
19. If (input1 is in1mf4) and (input2 is in2mf4) then (output is out1mf19) (1)
20. If (input1 is in1mf4) and (input2 is in2mf5) then (output is out1mf20) (1)
21. If (input1 is in1mf5) and (input2 is in2mf1) then (output is out1mf21) (1)
22. If (input1 is in1mf5) and (input2 is in2mf2) then (output is out1mf22) (1)
23. If (input1 is in1mf5) and (input2 is in2mf3) then (output is out1mf23) (1)
24. If (input1 is in1mf5) and (input2 is in2mf4) then (output is out1mf24) (1)
25. If (input1 is in1mf5) and (input2 is in2mf5) then (output is out1mf25) (1)

5.1.4.1.3 Merge Color Channel

For clinical Image (CT Image and MRI Image), yield of ANFIS is one segment vector that will be changed over into framework (size same as size of info Image) and in plain view as Image (Fused Image). In suit of shading Image (RGB), each shading channel input is applying to ANFIS independently; that is, for each pair of Images there are three one section vectors as yields from ANFIS. These yield vectors are changed over into lattices and at that point converge to frame Image (Fused Image). In this section we talk about the proposed technique and how it functions for the combination procedure. The strategy which is proposed has been tried tentatively and accomplished impressive and agreeable outcomes. The test results obtained through the present work is discussed in part 5.5.

5.1.5 Result and Discussion

In this section the outcome after execution is discussed and what has been carried out with respect to different images introduced. The significant geometrical highlights of shading Image and dim scale Image have been removed and coordinated with melded Image.

5.1.5.1 Simulation Result

Figure 5.13 show GUI through which client can without much of a stretch perform Image Combination task. This GUI created utilizing MATLAB. Here is information on Image pair chosen utilizing two press catches Select_image_1 and Select_Image_2. Intertwined Image press button used to combine the chosen Image. The chosen Image pair and Fused Image are shown in tomahawks.

Dataset: Multi-focus Image dataset gathered from http://dsp.etfbl.net/mif/.

PCA (Principle Component analysis): In Figure 5.14 the Image Combination is done on shading Image. PCA additionally gives practically proportionate outcome to ANFIS; yet, it shifts almost not at all in entropy and mean worth. The performance Analysis speaks to the worth which has been acquired for melded shading Images while applying both strategies. The significant contrast is that PCA is centred around the significant piece of the Image yet ANFIS works in all the pieces of the image (shown in Figure 5.15) .

5.1.5.2 Performance Analysis

Execution investigation of actualized model ANFIS and PCA has been done in term of mean and entropy.

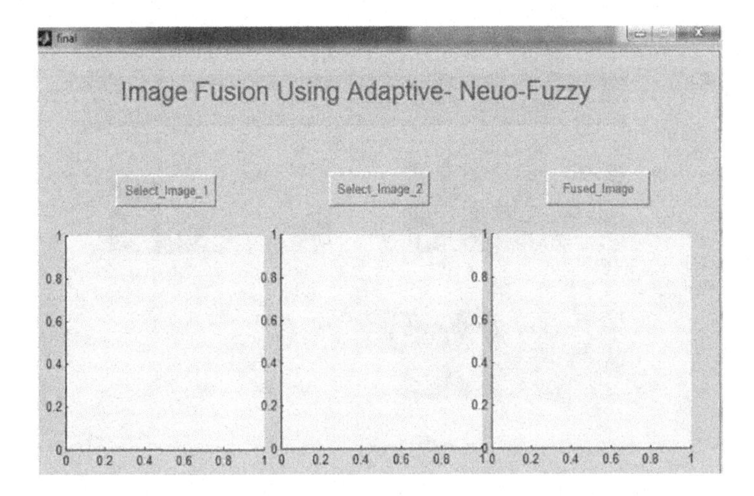

FIGURE 5.13 Image Fusion Using Adaptive Neuro Fuzzy.

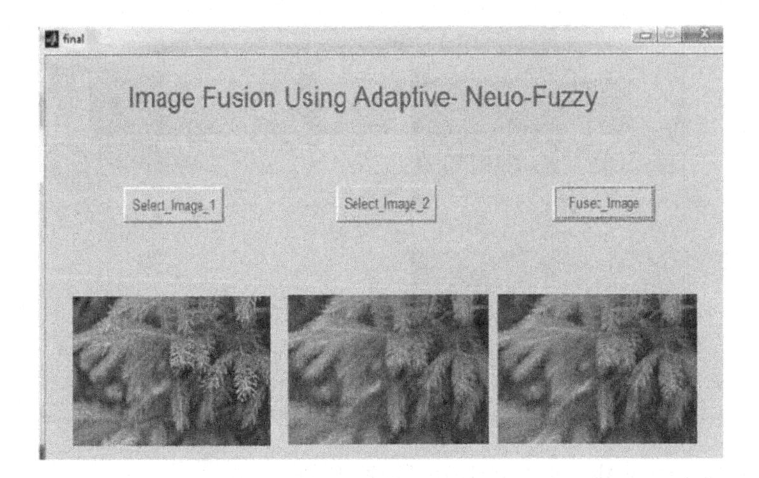

FIGURE 5.14 A Snapshot of Image Fusion (Fused Color Image Are Displayed).

The examination of both strategies—that is ANFIS based, and PCA based—analysed by utilizing the boundary known as entropy, and mean. Table 5.1 shows results determined from the two techniques are acceptable and palatable.

In the current section we discuss the outcome obtained in the current work. In this part, an information based model has been framed by thinking about the related highlights of shading Image as contextual analysis. It has been discovered that the created strategies in the current work are found to be agreeable.

5.1.6 Conclusion and Future Scope

A significant measure of work has been done on different images utilizing distinctive methodology. The current work has been completed for shading images and

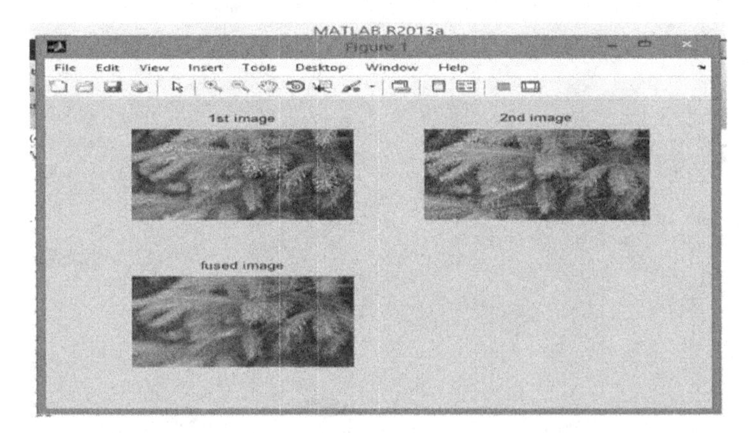

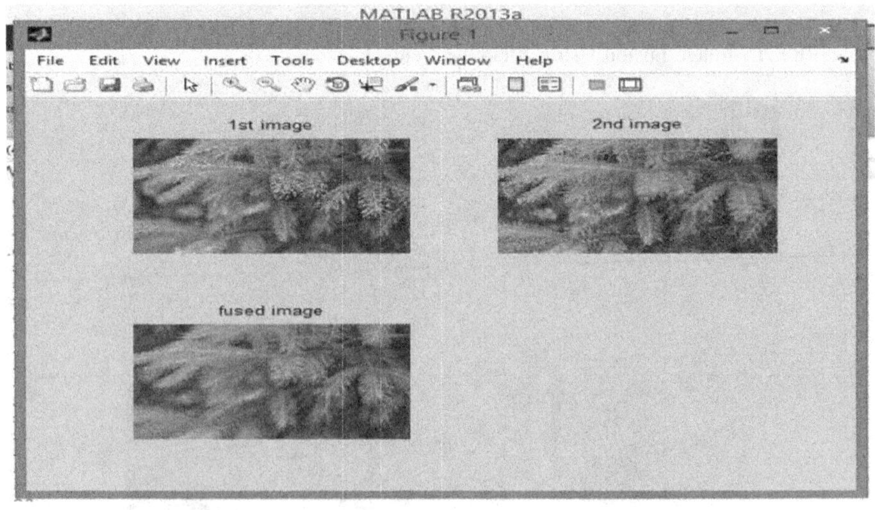

FIGURE 5.15 PCA Algorithm Apply for Fusing Color Image.

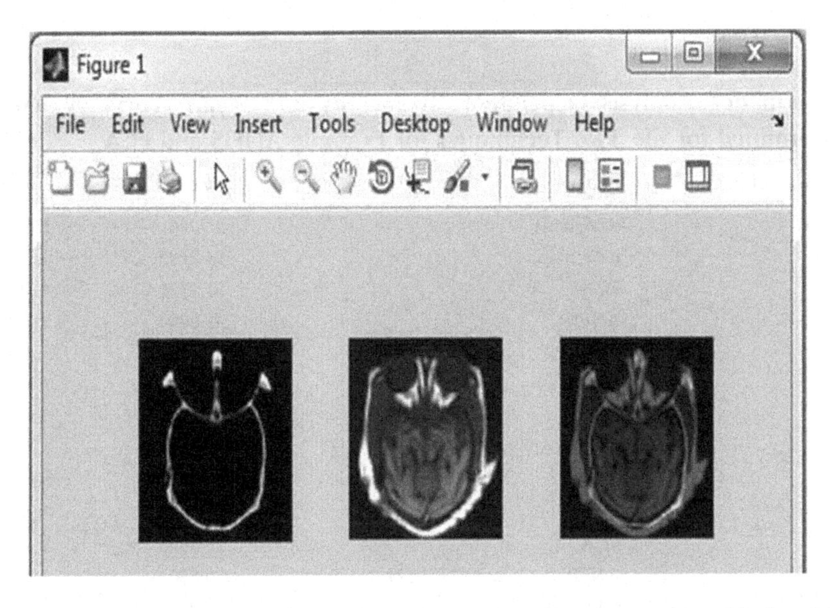

FIGURE 5.16 A Snap Shot CT and MRI Image Fusion (Fused Image Are Displayed for Grayscale Image or on Medical Image).

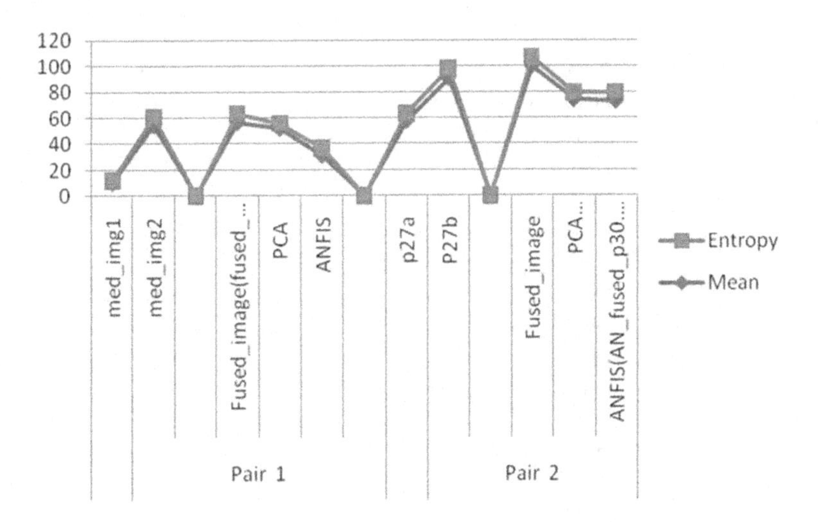

FIGURE 5.17 Performance Estimation in Medical and Shading Image of PCA and ANFIS.

clinical images utilizing Image Combination strategies. Versatile Neuro Fuzzy Inference System has been adjusted for study and examination of Image Combination for melding the assortment of Images. The commitments made in the section have been summed up and the extent of future work spelt out.

TABLE 5.1
Performance Analysis Dependent on Entropy and Mean Worth Which Is Determined for the Two Techniques for Example ANFIS and PCA

Experiment set	Images	Mean	Entropy
Pair 1	med_img1	9.9346	1.9247
	med_img2	54.2295	6.6325
	PCA	51.7376	4.1160
	ANFIS	31.0090	5.9541
	CT_1	57.4428	5.9577
Pair 2	MRI_1	90.4375	7.4750
	PCA	73.7856	5.3044
	ANFIS(AN_fused_CT_MRI_1.jpg)	72.3977	7.2537
	CT_2	65.0086	6.1814
Pair 3	MRI_2	76.1966	7.2999
	PCA	70.7966	5.2790
	ANFIS(An_fused_CT_MRI_2.jpg)	70.5307	7.2047
	CT_3	72.2441	6.8271
Pair 4	MRI_3	84.3076	7.5085
	PCA	76.1967	5.4060
	ANFIS	77.6928	7.4029
Pair 6	p27a	119.1838	6.4290
	P27b	121.5508	6.2747
	PCA (pca_fused_p27.jpg)	120.4096	6.3160
	ANFIS(AN_fused_p30.jpg)	120.2703	6.4848
	p30a	68.0190	6.1276
Pair 7	P30b	66.9919	6.0680
	PCA(pca_fused_p30.jpg)	67.5629	6.0912
	ANFIS(AN_fused_p30.jpg)	67.4527	6.2168
Pair 8	t3a	114.8771	7.8349
	t3b	126.2526	7.8530
	PCA(pca_fused_t3.jpg)	120.6586	7.8393
	ANFIS(An_fused_t3.jpg)	120.5280	7.8590
Pair 9	t4a	111.4796	7.5716
	t4b	119.3709	7.5627
	PCA	115.5654	7.5124
	ANFIS	115.3741	7.5228
Pair 10	t5a	88.8402	7.3739
	t5b	89.0884	7.3440
	PCA	88.9399	7.2342
	ANFIS	88.7996	7.2778
Pair 11	t6a	93.4168	7.1061
	t6b	94.2668	7.1941
	PCA	93.8637	7.0285
	ANFIS	93.6473	7.0520

(*Continued*)

TABLE 5.1 (Continued)
Performance Analysis Dependent on Entropy and Mean Worth Which Is Determined for the Two Techniques for Example ANFIS and PCA

Experiment set	Images	Mean	Entropy
Pair 12	t9a	68.6060	7.1062
	t9b	66.0645	7.0155
	PCA	67.3350	7.0986
	ANFIS	67.3282	7.1193
Pair 13	t28a	98.5045	7.5315
	t28b	106.2060	7.5559
	PCA	102.2884	7.4636
	ANFIS	102.1550	7.4829
Pair 14	t51a	87.8133	6.5017
	t51b	87.8964	6.4421
	PCA	87.8485	6.4233
	ANFIS	87.9773	6.5558
Pair 15	t58a	110.3165	6.7703
	t58b	110.7502	6.6148
	PCA	110.5456	6.6413
	ANFIS	110.4421	6.7464
Pair 16	t62a	104.6145	5.3714
	t62b	105.1041	5.1987
	PCA	104.7592	5.2566
	ANFIS	104.8334	5.3670
Pair 17	t63a	99.8076	5.6799
	t63b	99.5402	5.5064
	PCA	99.6643	5.4926
	ANFIS	99.7646	5.6218
Pair 18	t65a	66.5486	5.1910
	t65b	66.4747	5.2581
	PCA	66.5224	5.1570
	ANFIS	66.3100	5.1911
Pair 19	t70a	155.4721	7.0638
	t70b	154.0279	6.9512
	PCA	154.7800	6.9477
	ANFIS	154.7283	6.9902
Pair 20	t71a	188.9653	7.2277
	t71b	187.2606	7.3126
	PCA	188.0792	7.2883
	ANFIS	188.2019	7.2920
Pair 21	t72a	189.9532	7.0988
	t72b	192.6239	6.8845
	PCA	191.1244	6.9193
	ANFIS	191.3625	6.9399

In the current work ANFIS has been applied for combining the shading images. The work has been done in the accompanying stage: at the outset, we read the two-source shading Image from the same scene. At that point, we separated them into three channels; for example red, green and blue directs. In the next stage, we applied each channel to Adaptive Neuro Fuzzy Inference System. In the next stage consolidated or linked all the three channels. Finally, the conclusive outcome obtained was intertwined Image or one yield of the two-source Image; that is, integral data obtained from two Images is progressively enlightening and clearer.

Surgeon based Fuzzy Inference System executed to combine Image pair (clinical Images of CT and MRI and pair shading Image) The intertwined outcomes are generally obvious from the visual perspective. Agreeable entropy and means as contrasted and (PCA) Principal Component Analysis.

5.1.6.1 Future Scope

Pre-processing the data before mounding is conveyed in order to take out the anomalies. The ANFIS strategy must be entirely adaptable. It implies it works with present exploration issue as well as can be healthy for other examination issues moreover. The presentation investigation of ANFIS has been contrasted just and PCA strategy in the current work however in future it tends to be contrasted and other technique too.

REFERENCES

1. B. van Ginneken, C. M. Schaefer-Prokop, and M. Prokop, "Computer-aided diagnosis: how to move from the laboratory to the clinic", *Radiology*, vol. 261, no. 3, pp. 719–732, 2011.
2. S. Hu, E. A. Hoffman, and J. M. Reinhardt, "Automatic lung segmentation for accurate quantitation of volumetric X-ray CT images", *IEEE Transactions on Medical Imaging*, vol. 20, no. 6, pp. 490–498, 2001.
3. Q. Gao, S. J. Wang, D. Zhao, and J. Liu, "Accurate lung segmentation for X- ray CT images", in *Proceedings - Third International Conference on Natural Computation, ICNC 2007*, 2007, vol. 2, pp. 275–279.
4. Y. Wang, L. Liu, H. Zhang, Z. Cao, and S. Lu, "Image segmentation using active contours with normally biased GVF external force", *IEEE Signal Processing Letters*, vol. 17, no. 10, pp. 875–878, 2010.
5. T. F. Chan and L. A. Vese, "Active contours without edges", *IEEE Transactions on Image Processing*, vol. 10, no. 2, pp. 266–277, 2001.
6. W. Cui, Y. Wang, T. Lei, Y. Fan, and Y. Feng, "Local region statistics-based active contour model for medical image segmentation", in Proceedings - 2013 7th International Conference on Image and Graphics, ICIG 2013, 2013.
7. J. S. Athertya and G. S. Kumar, "Automatic initialization for segmentation of medical images based on active contour", in IECBES 2014, Conference Proceedings - 2014 IEEE Conference on Biomedical Engineering and Sciences: "Miri, Where Engineering in Medicine and Biology and Humanity Meet", 2015, pp. 446–451.
8. J. T. Pu, D. S. Paik, X. Meng, J. E. Roos, and G. D. Rubin, "Shape 'Break-and- Repair' strategy and its application to automated medical image segmentation", *IEEE Transactions Visualization Computer Graphics*, vol. 17, no. 1, pp. 115–124, 2011.
9. T. T. J. P. Kockelkorn, E. M. Van Rikxoort, J. C. Grutters, and B. Van Ginneken,

"Interactive lung segmentation in CT scans with severe abnormalities", in 2010 7th IEEE International Symposium on Biomedical Imaging: From Nano to Macro, ISBI 2010 - Proceedings, 2010, pp. 564–567.
10. A. Soliman *et al.*, "Accurate lungs segmentation on CT chest images by adaptive appearance-guided shape modeling", *IEEE Transactions on Medical Imaging*, vol. 36, no. 1, pp. 263–276, 2017.
11. S. Shen, A. A. T. Bui, J. Cong, and W. Hsu, "An automated lung segmentation approach using bidirectional chain codes to improve nodule detection accuracy", *Computers in Biology and Medicine*, vol. 57, pp. 139–149, 2015.
12. S. Zhou, Y. Cheng, and S. Tamura, "Automated lung segmentation and smoothing techniques for inclusion of juxtapleural nodules and pulmonary vessels on chest CT images", *Biomedical Signal Processing Control*, vol. 13, no. 1, pp. 62–70, 2014.
13. M. Orkisz, M. Hernández Hoyos, V. Pérez Romanello, C. Pérez Romanello, J.C. Prieto, and C. Revol-Muller, "Segmentation of the pulmonary vascular trees in 3D CT images using variational region-growing", *Innovation and Research in BioMedical Engineering*, vol. 35, no. 1, pp. 11–19, 2014.
14. B. Golosio *et al.*, "A novel multithreshold method for nodule detection in lung CT", *Medical Physics*, vol. 36, no. 8, pp. 3607–3618, 2009.
15. X. Ye, X. Lin, J. Dehmeshki, G. Slabaugh, and G. Beddoe, "Shape-based computer-aided detection of lung nodules in thoracic CT images", *IEEE Transactions on Biomedical Engineering*, vol. 56, no. 7, pp. 1810–1820, 2009.
16. M. Tan, R. Deklerck, B. Jansen, M. Bister, and J. Cornelis, "A novel computer-aided lung nodule detection system for CT images", *Medical Physics*, vol. 38, no. 10, pp. 5630–5645, 2011.
17. A. Teramoto *et al.*, "Hybrid method for the detection of pulmonary nodules using positron emission tomography/computed tomography: a preliminary study", *International Journal for Computer Assisted Radiology and Surgery*, vol. 9, no. 1, pp. 59–69, 2014.
18. M. S. Brown *et al.*, "Toward clinically usable CAD for lung cancer screening with computed tomography", *European Radiology*, vol. 24, no. 11, pp. 2719–2728, 2014.
19. H. Han, L. Li, F. Han, B. Song, W. Moore, and Z. Liang, "Fast and adaptive detection of pulmonary nodules in thoracic CT images using a hierarchical vector quantization scheme", *IEEE Journal of Biomedical and Health Informatics*, vol. 19, no. 2, pp. 648–659, 2015.
20. X. Liu, F. Hou, H. Qin, and A. Hao, "A CADe system for nodule detection in thoracic CT images based on artificial neural network", *Science China Information Sciences*, vol. 60, no. 7, pp. 1–15, 2017.
21. K. Clark *et al.*, "The cancer imaging archive (TCIA): maintaining and operating a public information repository", Journal of Digital Imaging, vol. 26, no. 6, pp. 1045–1057, 2013.
22. Shukla S., Raja R., "A survey on fusion of color images", ISSN: 2278 – 1323 International Journal of Advanced Research in Computer Engineering & Technology (IJARCET), vol. 5, no. 6, pp. 287–300, June 2016.
23. Shukla S., Rohit R., "Digital image fusion using adaptive neuro-Fuzzy inference system, International Journal of New Technology and Research (IJNTR) ISSN:2454-4116, vol. 2, no. 5, pp. 101–104, May 2016.
24. M. Firmino, G. Angelo, H. Morais, M. R. Dantas, and R. Valentim, "Computer-aided detection (CADe) and diagnosis (CADx) system for lung cancer with likelihood of malignancy", *BioMedical Engineering OnLine*, vol. 15, no. 1, pp. 1–17, 2016.
25. J. kui Liu *et al.*, "An assisted diagnosis system for detection of early pulmonary nodule in computed tomography images", *Journal of Medical Systems*, vol. 41, no. 2, 2017.
26. E. Taşcı and A. Uğur, "Shape and texture based novel features for automated

juxtapleural nodule detection in lung CTs", *Journal of Medical Systems*, vol. 39, no. 5, pp. 1–13, 2015.

27. A. O. de Carvalho Filho, W. B. de Sampaio, A. C. Silva, A. C. de Paiva, R. A. Nunes, and M. Gattass, "Automatic detection of solitary lung nodules using qualitythreshold clustering, genetic algorithm and diversity index", *Artificial Intelligence in Medicine*, pp. 165–177,Vol. 1, 2013.
28. W. J. Choi and T. S. Choi, "Automated pulmonary nodule detection based on three-dimensional shape-based feature descriptor", *Computer Methods and Programs in Biomedicine*, vol. 113, no. 1, pp. 37–54, 2014.
29. J. Kuruvilla and K. Gunavathi, "Lung cancer classification using neural networks for CT images", Computer Methods and Programs in Biomedicine, vol. 113, no. 1, pp. 202–209, 2013.
30. R. Golan, C. Jacob, and J. Denzinger, "Lung nodule detection in CT images using deep convolutional neural networks", *IJCNN International Joint Conference on Neural Networks*, no. 1, pp. 243–250, 2016.
31. M. Alilou, V. Kovalev, E. Snezhko, and V. Taimouri, "A comprehensive framework for automatic detection of pulmonary nodules in lung CT images", *Image Analysis and Stereology*, vol. 33, no. 1, pp. 13–27, 2014.
32. S. G. Armato, and W. F. Sensakovic, "Automated lung segmentation for thoracic CT: impact on computer-aided diagnosis", Academic Radiology, vol. 11, no. 9, pp. 1011–1021, 2004.
33. M. Keshani, Z. Azimifar, F. Tajeripour, and R. Boostani, "Lung nodule segmentation and recognition using SVM classifier and active contour modeling: a complete intelligent system", Computers in Biology and Medicine, vol. 43, no. 4, pp. 287–300, 2013.

6 Medical Imaging in Healthcare Applications

K. Rawal, G. Sethi, and D. Ghai

CONTENTS

6.1 INTRODUCTION

Medical image processing is an important tool for diagnosis and prognosis of disease. However, with the increased volume of digital data, the demand for accuracy and efficiency in medical image processing techniques is also increasing. With the help of medical imaging and recent advancements in artificial intelligence, researchers are able to develop a Computer Aided Diagnostic system (CAD) for the characterization of the diseases. With the advent of the latest and most advanced image technologies, physicians are now able to visualize the hidden details in medical images. Thus, computer aids are not only required but have become indispensable in the physician's diagnostic process. Computerized systems can be employed to assist physicians in the diagnosis of diseases at early stages and hence reduce the dependency on invasive methods for the purpose of diagnosis [1, 2]. However, there are many disadvantages that are associated with CT and MRI. CT scan is best for bone injuries, chest related diseases and the detection of tumors in the abdomen. On the other hand, MRI is suitable for examining soft tissues and brain tumors. The CT scan takes approximately 5 minutes, but MRIs can takes up to 30 minutes. In the case of CT, there is a risk of exposure to radiation, but MRI does not use ionized radiations. CT scan does not cause claustrophobia, but MRI often does. Moreover, CT scan is cheaper in cost compared to the MRI. These advantages make the CT scan an attractive candidate for imaging the abdomen for the diagnosis of disease.

6.2 IMAGE MODALITIES

The most prevalent image modalities are reviewed as follows:-

6.2.1 PET Scan

The Positron Emission Tomography (PET) scan generates an image that captures the chemical changes in tissues [3].

The PET scanner is shown below in Figure 6.1. It is an imaging technique for examining physiological activities. The PET makes use of shortlived radioactive materials to produce high quality images. The tracer amounts are determined quantitatively, thus making PET imaging an ideal candidate for biomedical applications. The PET images found applications in oncology, cardiology and diseases related to the artery. The PET image of the abdomen is shown below in Figure 6.2.

The material injected into the body of the patient is a combination of sugar and radioactive material. The scan shows the functioning of organs and tissues within the body by absorbing sugar and further detects the radioactive material that the computer translates into the image [3]. This is considered the most effective type of nuclear medicine procedures for diagnosis of disease. But there are disadvantages that make this technology inaccessible to the average patient.

The machinery related to PET scans is still not available in many hospitals in India because of the prohibitive cost involved. The biggest disadvantage is the danger of exposing the patient to radiation. The radiation is dangerous to the patient in the case of continuous exposure.

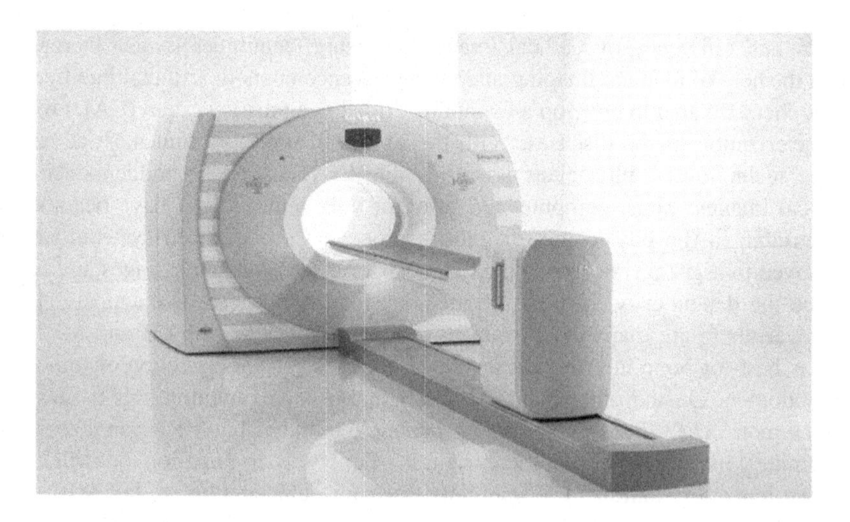

FIGURE 6.1 Siemen's PET Scanner (Image Source: http://www.healthcare.siemens.com/) [3].

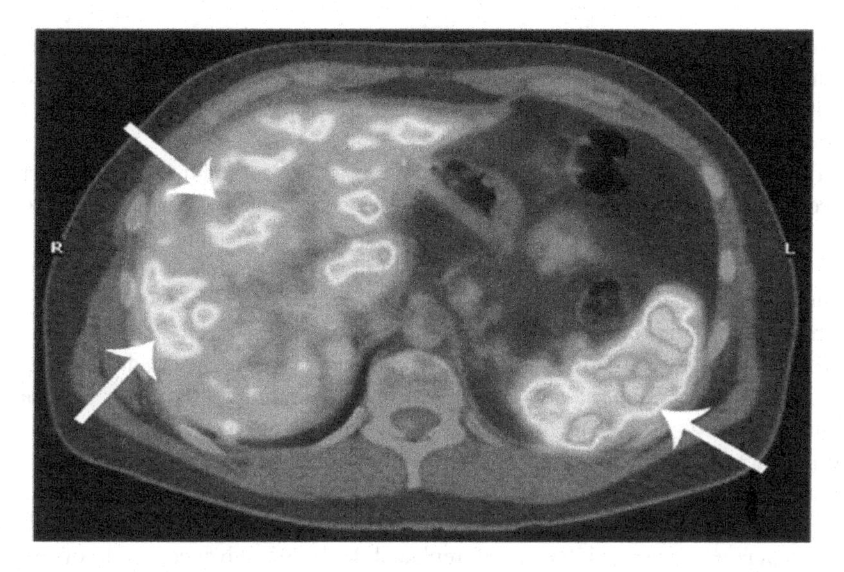

FIGURE 6.2 PET Image of the Abdomen (Image Source: http://www.Clinicalimagingscience.org/) [4].

6.2.2 Ultrasound

Ultrasound imaging is considered one of the most popular image modalities. The ultrasound equipment is available in almost all hospitals. The ultrasound image of the abdomen is shown in Figure 6.3 [5]. It works on the principle of emission of sound waves having a frequency greater than the audible frequency range. The

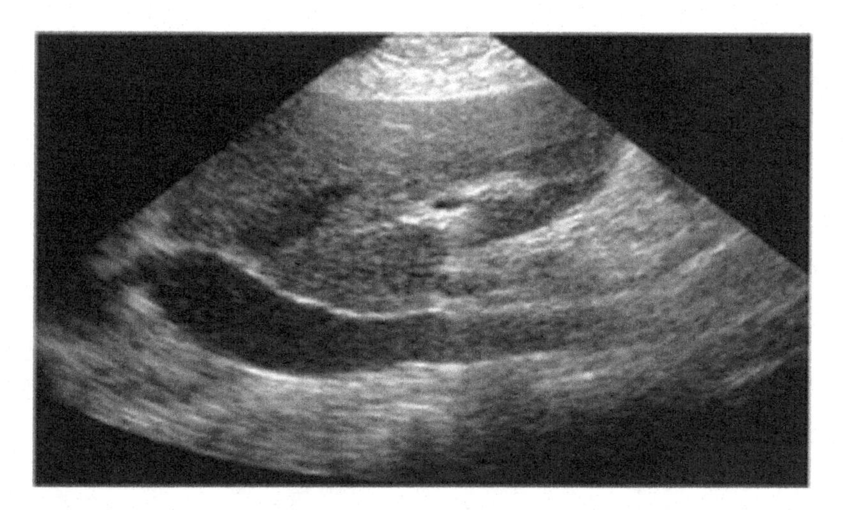

FIGURE 6.3 Ultrasound Image of the Abdomen (Image Source http://www.jefferson.edu/university/) [7].

frequency range varies from 2 to 15 MHz. At this frequency range, the velocity of sound waves within the patient's body is close to 1540 m/s [6]. The well-known application of ultrasound is sonography. It is used for the purpose of screening. The ultrasound system is shown in Figure 6.4.

The procedure of performing sonography consists of a hand-held probe which is placed directly on the body of the patient. By moving the probe—, i.e., transducer —over the body of the patient, an ultrasound image appears on the monitor.

The disadvantage of ultrasound is the inability to reduce false positives, leading to unnecessary and painful biopsies, especially in the case of abdominal diseases such as tumors that may not be detected by ultrasound correctly. Abdominal diseases will not be straightforward in their ultrasound appearance and thus, the ultrasound images are not always conclusive in their findings. Moreover, ultrasound equipment needs regular upgrades and servicing to make the equipment ready to work. Ultrasound is considered one of the most important medical imaging modalities for the purpose of diagnosis. The speckle noise in ultrasound imaging corrupts the output, thereby preventing accurate observation. Thus, due to these disadvantages ultrasound has been replaced by more advanced state-of-the-art image modalities like CT and MRI.

6.2.3 MRI Scan

Magnetic and radio waves are used for creating an image of the inside of the body parts in the MRI scan. These waves further create cross-sectional images of the abdomen which enable the specialist to check for tissue and organ abnormalities without making an opening over the body; hence avoiding the need for biopsies for

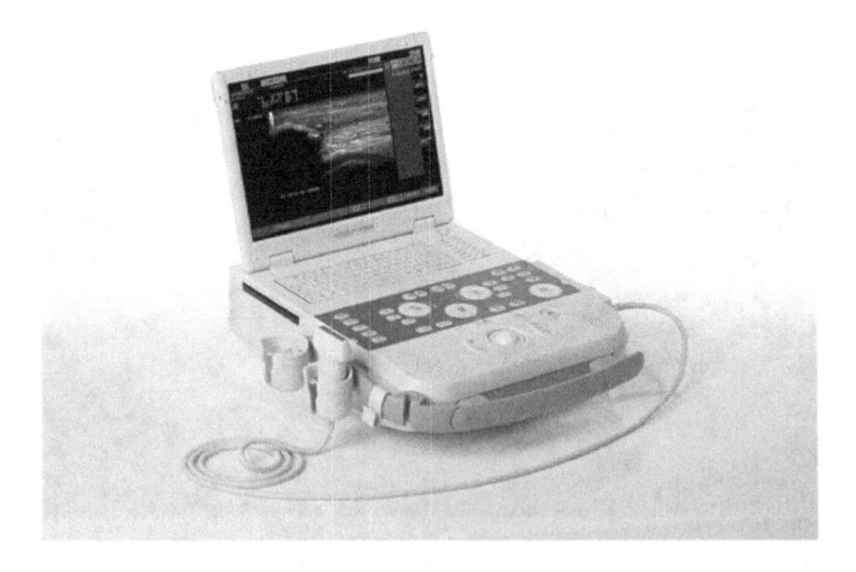

FIGURE 6.4 Ultrasound System (Image Source: http://www.healthcare.siemens.com/) [3].

diagnosis of diseases [4]. Unlike X-rays, thge MRI scan does not use radiation. The MRI image of the abdomen is shown below in Figure 6.5.

Magnetic resonance imaging can provide specific tissue characterization and hence provide a very specific diagnosis. The typical MRI system is shown below in Figure 6.6. The abdominal MRI provides detailed images of the belly area, as shown in Figure 6.7. The MRI test can be used to look at the flow of blood, causes of swelling and pain in the abdomen, abnormal flow of blood that causes liver and kidney problems and masses in the liver, kidneys or spleen. MRI, unlike X-rays and CT scans, does not use any radiation for the diagnosis of disease.

This is the biggest advantage of the noninvasive technique of image modality popularly known as MRI. However, the principle of high magnetic radiation, upon which it operates, can cause heart pacemakers or defibrillation devices to malfunction [4]. Moreover, the expensive equipment inflates the cost of the MRI scan.

The scan is generally done in closed areas, so patients may encounter the problem of claustrophobia. The MRI scanner involves loud noises because of the high amount of current involved in the input supply. The limitations of MRI scans include cost, availability of equipment, especially in enhanced MR imaging, and the inability to differentiate intermediate fibrosis.

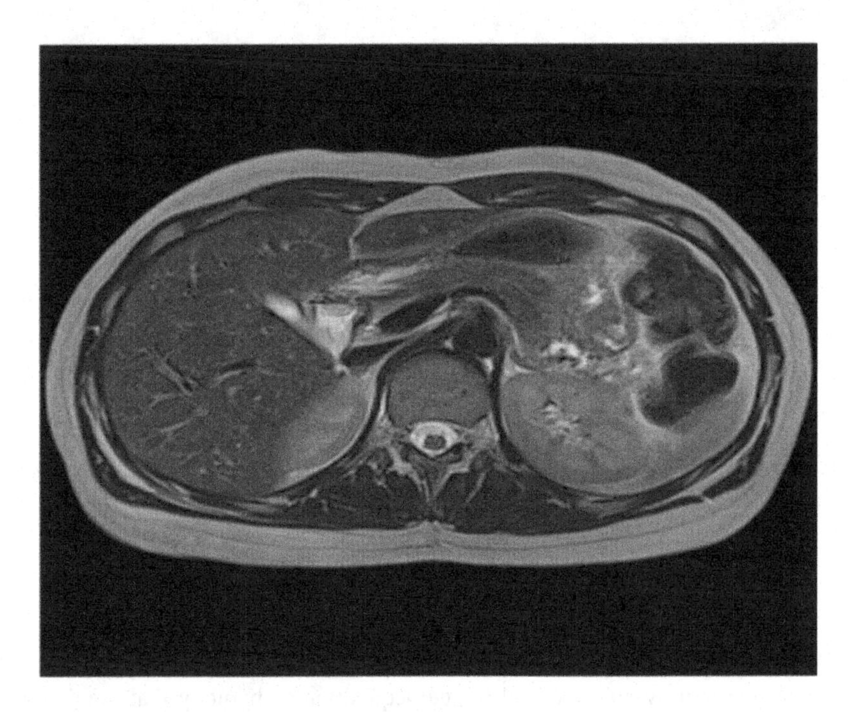

FIGURE 6.5 MRI Image of the Abdomen (Image Source: http://doveimaging.co/) [8].

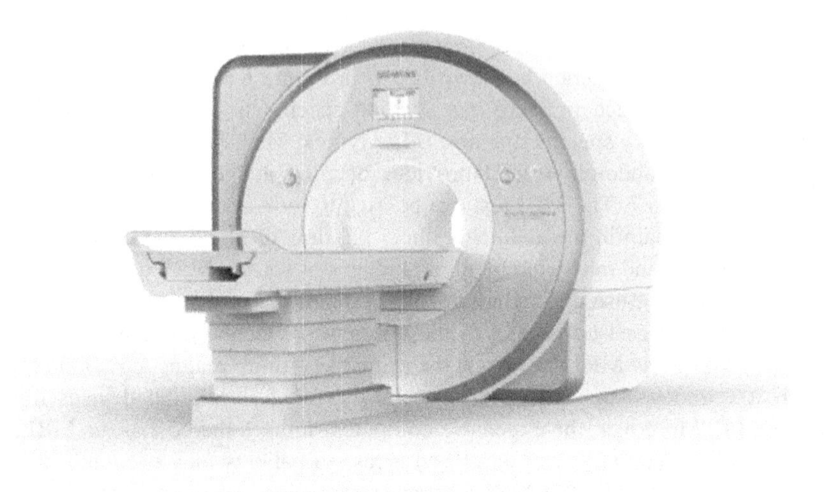

FIGURE 6.6 MRI Scanner (Image Source: http://www.healthcare.siemens.com/) [3].

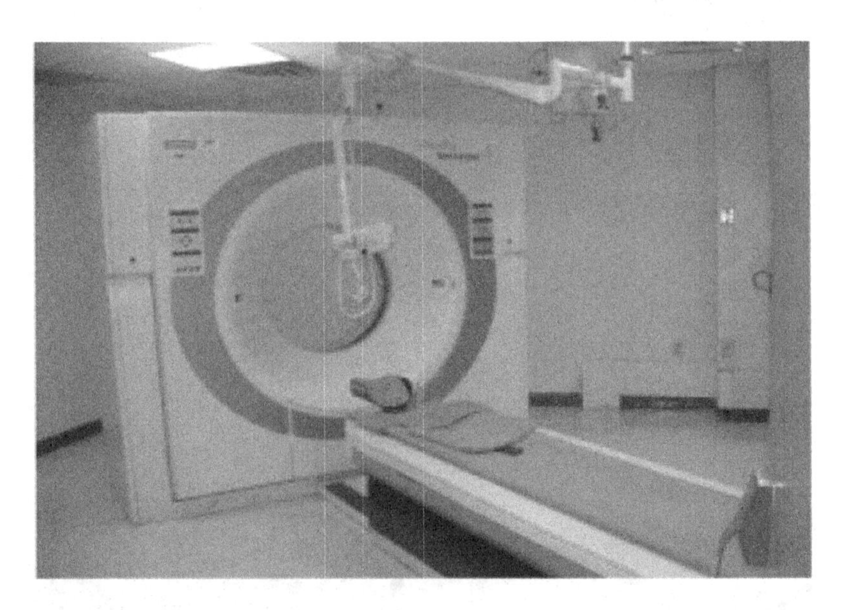

FIGURE 6.7 CT Scanner (Image Source: http://www.healthcare.siemens.com/) [3].

6.2.4 CT Scan

CT scan is a noninvasive medical image acquisition technology that requires external contrast to find optimal results. The typical CT scanner is shown below in Figure 6.8. It uses X-ray equipment from different angles around the body and shows the cross-section view of the body organs. The specialist can confirm the

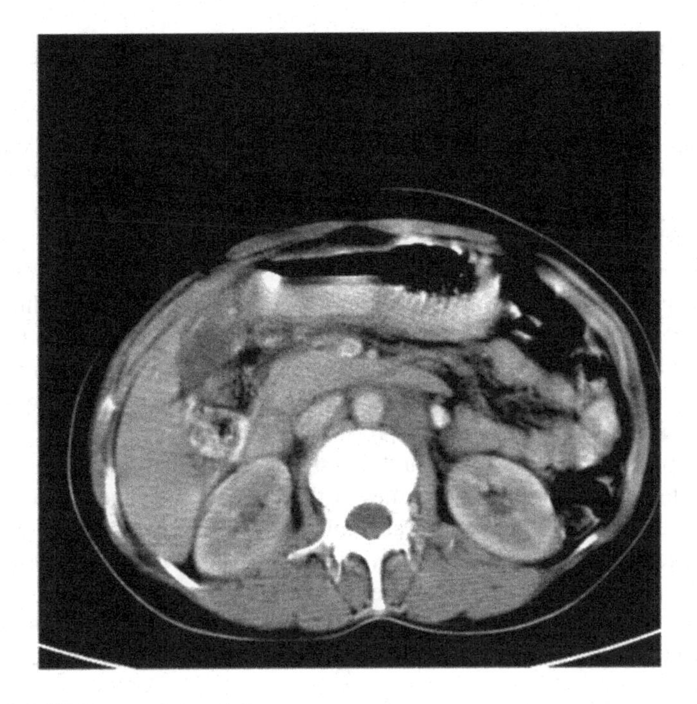

FIGURE 6.8 CT Image of the Abdomen.

presence of disease by interpreting the scan of the organ and also comment on the extent of the spread of disease across the organ [4].

The accuracy of CT is increased with high imaging speed that makes them the perfect candidate for high speed applications of medical image processing. CT scans remain the best modality option in case of abdominal diseases like liver tumors even if MRI may offer slightly better results in some cases [9]. The typical Abdominal CT scan is shown below in Figure 6.8. Following are the advantages of CT scan:

- CT scan is painless and noninvasive in nature.
- CT images gives detailed and precise view sof abdominal organs far better than conventional X-ray imaging.
- The process of CT scanning is fast.
- In emergency situations, CT detects internal injuries also.
- The CT scan has been a cost-effective tool for a variety of clinical applications.

6.3 RECENT TRENDS IN HEALTHCARE TECHNOLOGY

Human health is significantly improved by using the recent advancements in healthcare technologies. Various technologies in medical imaging, like computer assisted image processing leads to the early diagnosis of disease. The increased volume of data of medical images like CT, MRI and Ultrasound placing a huge diagnostic burden on radiologists. In this context, the computerized diagnostic systems will accentuate the diagnostic accuracy, reduce cost and increase efficiency.

Diseases related to the abdomen are prevalent all over the world because of the lack of basic facilities like clean water, nutritious food, contaminated food and a sedentary living style. The commonly known abdominal diseases are related to the liver, kidney and gall bladder. In recent years, digital imaging data has increased tremendously and outnumbered the availability of the radiologists. This increase in workload directly impacts the performance of the radiologists. Therefore, human analysis is not in harmony with the quantum of the data to be handled. Thus, there is a need to develop a computer assisted texture analysis and classification framework to assist radiologists in dealing with such a huge amount of data. Moreover, it is difficult to design the CAD by using the texture information because the gray level intensities are overlapping in nature [10–17].

Designing an accurate, efficient and robust computer aided diagnostic framework for characterization of abdomen tissues is the biggest challenge faced by the researchers because representation of abdominal tissues are overlapping in nature.

In addition, accuracy is insufficiently high to use these diagnostic systems commercially. Therefore, there is a strong need to design a diagnostic framework that can characterize abdominal tissues like tumor, cysts, stone and normal tissues accurately and efficiently. The various building blocks of the diagnostic framework are as follows:

1. Image segmentation
2. Feature extraction
3. Feature selection
4. Feature classification

6.4 SCOPE FOR FUTURE WORK

The involvement of computers is indispensible in diagnosing medical images. The increased volume of medical data leads to the development of the computer-aided diagnosis systems which further improves the accuracy and efficiency of radiologists in diagnosing various diseases. An effort is already made by various researchers to design a diagnostic framework for characterization of abdominal tissues which is highly accurate and is able to characterize multiple abdomen tissues [18–24]. However, there are still a number of issues that need to be addressed to make computer aided diagnosis more commercially visible. Following are the issues needs to be addressed:-

1. Several systems have already been designed for characterization of abdominal tissues in CT images based on their texture properties. More abdomen diseases can be added based on shape features like pancreatitis.
2. Efforts are required to make computer aided diagnostic frameworks more accurate, reliable and invariant to changes in illumination, rotation, and size of CT image.
3. The segmentation method proposed until now are semi-automatic in nature. Manual interventions are still required in the segmentation methods proposed by various authors to create the edge map. Efforts are required to reduce

manual intervention, and automatic methods are needed to improves diagnostic accuracy.
4. In the features selection stage, the flexi scale curvelet transform is used for optimizing curvelet features by selecting an appropriate scale using an improved genetic algorithm.
5. The finding of the methods proposed in this area can be used for hardware implementation of CAD that can be integrated with the CT scanner.
6. Machine learning algorithms can also be used to automate the process of tuning of controlling parameters. The automation process can be done using some priories taken from the segmented ROIs. The machine learning algorithm can initially check the conditions that are required to fix the controlling parameters; then based on the prior knowledge, the controlling parameters can be tuned. As far as implementation on hardware is concerned, the variable parameters approach based on clinical context must be used instead of fixed tuning parameters in order to get the desirable results [25–27].
7. The other future enhancements would be to incorporate the latest technologies like nanotechnology etc., into the CAD system for better performance of the system.

6.5 CONCLUSIONS

The process of diagnosing abdominal diseases is a challenging and tedious task for any physician.The hHigh morbidity rate of abdominal diseases has been observed and thus there is a need for diagnosis at an early stage to avoid the use of invasive methods. However, the large amount of data along with the subjectivity of examining diseases significantly affects the diagnostic results. Developments in this field are evolving continuously, providing significant improvement in medical image processing and classification. The work done in this field would also make a contribution to noninvasive diagnosis of abdomen diseases and constitute an effort in the direction of providing effective healthcare.

REFERENCES

1. C. Choi, "The current status of imaging diagnosis of hepatocellular carcinoma," Liver Transplantation, vol. 10, no 2, pp. S20–S25, 2004.
2. R. Freeman, A. Mithoefer, R. Ruthazer, K. Nguyen, A. Schore, A. Harper, and E. Edwards, "Optimizing staging for hepatocellular tumor before liver transplantation: a retrospective analysis of the UNOS/OPTN database," *American Association for the Study of Liver Diseases, Liver Transplantation*, vol. 12, no 10, pp. 1504–1511, 2006.
3. http://www.health care.siemens.com/.
4. http://www. Clinicalimagingscience.org/.
5. http://www.jefferson.edu/university/.
6. J. Jensen, "*Medical Ultrasound Imaging*," Elsevier Ltd., 2006.
7. http://www.jefferson.edu/university/.
8. http://doveimaging.co/.
9. D. Pescia, "Segmentation of liver tumors on CT images," Ph. D. Thesis, France, Ecole Centrale Paris, 2011.
10. G. Sethi, B. S. Saini, and D. Singh, "Segmentation of cancerous regions in liver using

an edge based and phase congruent region enhancement method," *Computer and Electrical Engineering*, Elsevier, vol. 46, pp. 78–96, 2015.
11. G. Sethi, and B. S. Saini, "Computer aided diagnosis using flexi-scale curvelet transform using improved genetic algorithm," *Australasian Physical & Engineering Sciences in Medicine*, Springer, vol. 38, no. 4, pp. 671–688, 2015.
12. G. Sethi, and B. S. Saini, "Segmentation of abdomen diseases using active contours in CT images," *Biomedical Engineering: Application Basis and Communication*, World Scientific, vol. 27, pp. 1550047–1550054, 2015.
13. Q. Aureline, M. Ingrid, H. Denis, S. Gerard, and P. William, "Assessing the classification of liver focal lesions by using multi-phase computer tomography scans," *Medical Content-Based Retrieval for Clinical Decision Support*, vol. 7723, pp. 80–91, 2013.
14. S. Mougiakakou, I. Valavanis, N. Mouravliansky, and K. Nikita, "DIiagnosis: a telematics-enabled system for medical image archiving, management, and diagnosis assistance," *IEEE Transactions on Instrumentation and Measurement*, vol. 58, pp. 2113–2120, 2009.
15. U. Mei, T. Tomoko, K. Shinya, T. Hidetoshi, H. Xian-Hua, K. Shuzo, F. Akira, and C. Yen-Wei, "Statistical shape model of the liver and its application to computer-aided diagnosis of liver cirrhosis," *Electrical Engineering in Japan*, vol. 190, pp. 37–45, 2014.
16. G. Balasubramanian, and S. Natesan, "Computer-aided diagnosis system for classifying benign and malignant thyroid nodules in multi-stained FNAB cytological images," *Australasian Physical & Engineering Sciences in Medicine*, vol. 36, pp. 219–230, 2013.
17. S. Kumar, R. Moni, and J. Rajeesh, "An automatic computer-aided diagnosis system for liver tumors on computed tomography images," *Computer and Electrical Engineering*, vol. 39, pp. 1516–1526, 2013.
18. A. Aaron, R. Daniel, and C. Gunnar, "Classification of hepatic lesions using the matching metric," *Journal of Computer Vision and Image Understanding*, vol. 121, pp. 36–42, 2014.
19. D. E. Goldberg, "Genetic algorithms in search optimization and machine Learning," Addison-Wesley, Boston, 1988.
20. D. Whitley, T. Starkweather, and C. Bogart, "Genetic algorithms and neural networks: optimizing connections and connectivity," *Parallel Computing*, vol. 14, pp. 347–361, 1990.
21. M. Keki, "A unified explanation for the adaptive capacity of simple recombinative genetic algorithms," Ph. D. Thesis, Computer Science Department, Brandeis Universit, 2009.
22. R. Larry, "Multi-objective site selection and analysis for GSM cellular network planning," Ph. D. Thesis, Cardiff University, 2005.
23. T. Deselaers, T. Weyand, and H. Ney, "Image retrieval and annotation using maximum entropy," *In Proceedings CLEF 2006, Springer, Lecture Notes in Computer Science (LNCS)*, vol. 4730, pp 725–734, 2006.
24. T. Deselaers, H. Muller, P. Clough, H. Ney, and T. M. Lehmann, "The CLEF 2005 automatic medical image annotation task," *International Journal of Computer Vision*, vol. 74, pp. 51–58, 2007.
25. U. Avni, J. Goldberger, and H. Greenspan, "Tau MIPLAB at Image Clef 2008," *In Working Notes of CLEF 2008*, Aarhus, Denmark, 2008.
26. L. Setia, A. Teynor, A. Halawani, and H. Burkhardt, "Grayscale medical image annotation using local relational features," *Pattern Recognition Letters*, vol. 29, pp. 2039–2045, 2008.
27. T. Tommasi, F. Orabona, and B. Caputo, "CLEF 2007 image annotation task: an SVM–based cue integration approach," Proceedings of Image CLEF 2007 -LNCS, *in Working Notes of CLEF 2007*, Budapest, Hungary, 2007.

7 Classification of Diabetic Retinopathy by Applying an Ensemble of Architectures

Rahul Hooda and Vaishali Devi

CONTENTS

7.1 INTRODUCTION

Diabetes is one of the most widespread diseases with complications affecting numerous systems in the body [1]. Every year there are millions of new patients diagnosed with diabetes. The global prevalence of the disease is also increasing with each year [2]. Persons with a historical presence of diabetes are also prone to an aftereffect known as diabetic retinopathy. Diabetic retinopathy (DR) is a disease generated as an effect of diabetes that harms the eyes of the patient. DR happens in patients who have high sugar levels in their blood. As a consequence of diabetes, tiny blood vessels in the retina become blocked. DR is induced by the destruction of light-sensitive tissue present in blood vessels at the back of the eye. Damaged blood vessels cause a blood shortage in the region of the retina and can lead to long-lasting loss of eyesight . There is no initial sign of this disease and it can often be diagnosed only when the patient starts to lose vision. The effect of diabetic retinopathy varies from mild vision problems to complete blindness.

In persons with diabetes, the presence of retinopathy in India is about 18%. Most of the guidelines recommend annual screening of diabetic patients, even if they have no symptoms of retinopathy. Early diagnosis of this disease can be possible only through regular screening and monitoring. Proper screening of DR aids in initial detection, proper cure and a reduction in the probability of developing full blindness. Manual screening is not feasible since either patients have to come to health centres or doctors have to reach out to them. Classification of diabetic retinopathy involves assigning weight to different features and the location of these features by expert doctors. This process consumes a lot of the doctor's time, and also sometimes that of the patient, who due to ignorance, fear or carelessness arrives at the hospital at such a late stage that it became difficult to save their eyes. Thus, computer-aided diagnosis (CAD) systems need to be developed for automatic classification of diabetic retinopathy. CAD system for the unmasking of DR takes fundus images as input. These fundus images are also used to diagnose many other eye diseases. Some of the CAD systems developed have the scope to differentiate between normal and anomalous retinal images. These systems are supposed to decrease the assigned work of the eye specialist by rejecting the healthy images with the help of the CAD system.

In this paper, an ensemble is presented that combines the results of three different standard architectures to segregate the fundus images into healthy images and images having DR. In Section 2, the work done in the space of classification of DR is discussed. In Section 3, the presented method and the dataset used are outlined. In Section 4, the outcome obtained from different architectures and ensembles are presented. Lastly, the findings are summarized in Section 5.

7.1.1 Literature Survey

In the literature, different methods have been presented to classify and detect retinopathy in fundus images.

Ege et al. [3] presented a technique for diagnosis of diabetic retinopathy in which different statistical classifiers are tested. The tested classifiers includes Bayesian, Mahalanobis and KNN classifier. Out of the three classifiers, Mahalanobis classifier gave the best result.

Sinthanayothin et al. [4] discussed a method in which the principal parts of the retina are automatically detected. Then different features are extracted to identify the hard exudates, hemorrhages and microaneurysms. All the extracted features are used to conclude whether diabetic retinopathy is present or not.

Vallabha et al. [5] used vascular abnormalities to automatically classify diabetic retinopathy. To detect vascular abnormalities, selective Gabor filters were used. The output obtained from these features is used to classify the fundus image as moderate or severe case of diabetic retinopathy.

Sopharak et al. [6] presented a method to identify exudates, which is the dominant indication of diabetic retinopathy, from the digital images. Different features like standard deviation, intensity, edge pixels and hue are extracted to form a feature vector. These features are provided as input to FCM clustering method which provide detection results. These result are compared with the results provided by expert ophthalmologists.

Gulshan et al. [7] applied a multi-layered CNN algorithm to automatically classify diabetic retinopathy and macular edema. To detect diabetic retinopathy, two different datasets, namely Messidor dataset and EyePACS dataset have been used. The results indicate that the presented algorithm has high specificity and sensitivity for the two diseases. The results need further validation before applying the algorithm in clinical settings.

Amin et al. [8] presented an automatic technique for classification and detection of exudates using fundus images. In this four main descriptors are used to choose the feature group for each candidate lesion. Combinations of different classifiers are tested and the best combination is used to enhance the performance of the system. The presented technique is compared with the existing methods using accuracy measure and area under the curve (AUC) measure. It is concluded that the suggested method outperform all the current methodologies.

Li et al. [9] applied transfer learning using CNN to classify retinal fundus images for diabetic retinopathy. To perform experiments two publicly available datasets namely DR1 and MESSIDOR has been used. In this different experiments have been performed in which pre-trained models are directly used as well as fine-tuning is also performed. The results proved that transfer learning improves the result as well as the performance of CNN models to classify diabetic retinopathy.

Xu et al. [10] explored the application of deep learning to reveal diabetic retinopathy using colored retinal fundus images. In this paper, a modified CNN network is used for the segregation and the accuracy of 94.5% is achieved.

Gargeya and Leng [11] proposed a deep learning algorithm that is data driven and automatically detects diabetic retinopathy. In this, 75137 publicly available fundus images are used for the purpose of testing and training. The developed model achieved 0.97 AUC using 5-fold cross verification method. The achieved performance suggests that the proposed method is highly reliable.

Akram et al. [12] developed a system comprising of unique hybrid classifier for the finding of lesions in the retina, which ultimately helps in the grading of diabetic retinopathy. In this system, after pre-processing, all the regions are detected which may have candidate lesions. For every contender region, a descriptor set is created using shape, intensity and statistics features. Hybrid classifier, combining Gaussian Mixture Model and m-Mediods based modeling approach, is used to enhance the grading accuracy. The architecture performance is measured using different specifiers such as accuracy, AUC, specificity and sensitivity. It achieved the AUC performance 0.981 which is superior than the individual methods.

Pratt et al. [13] also presented a CNN method to distinguish retinal fundus images for DR. In this, a publicly available Kaggle dataset is used and on this dataset, data augmentation is performed to enhance the medical dataset. The method achieved the validation accuracy of 75%. The images have been classified into five different classes.

Dutta et al. [14] proposed an automatic knowledge model in which key features are identified that can suggest the beginning of diabetic retinopathy. The proposed model is trained using three Neural networks (NN); namely back propagation NN, deep NN and convolutional NN. It is experimentally obtained that deep learning-based NN performs better than back propagation NN.

Wan et al. [15] presented an automatic technique to detect DR by applying CNN. The method works in three different fields of segmentation, detection and classification. Different CNN models namely AlexNet, VGGNet, GoogleNet and ResNet have been fine-tuned and analyzed. The greatest classification accuracy achieved by these models is 95.68%.

Zhao and Hamarneh [16] presented a method to enhance the deep learning based classifiers in analyzing retinal fundus images. The authors used prior knowledge about the vessels structures related to diabetic retinopathy. A dual layer LSTM module is also used to grasp the dependencies between different vessel structures. The authors claim that the proposed method enhances the performance up to 8%.

Rehman et al. [17] used a deep learning approach for diabetic retinopathy classification. The authors tested pre-trained CNN models, as well as a customized CNN model for this purpose. The best accuracy of 98.15% has been achieved on customized CNN.

7.2 METHOD AND DATA

7.2.1 Dataset Used

In medical image analysis, a major hurdle in the development of CAD systems is the lack of publicly available datasets. For diabetic retinopathy, IDRiD dataset is publicly accessible. IDRiD stands for Indian Diabetic Retinopathy Image Dataset and it is the first dataset of DR that is based on the Indian public. The dataset was released as a segment of "Diabetic Retinopathy: Segmentation and Grading Challenge" regulated in partnership with IEEE [18]. The dataset contains 516 colored images of retinal fundus. The images are in.jpg format. The dataset contains images of two types that are retinal images with proof of retinopathy (abnormal images) and without proof of retinopathy (normal images). The dataset contains ground truth in which each image is graded between 0 (normal) and 4 (severe diabetic retinopathy). These images have been graded by expert medical experts. In this paper, images have been classified into 2 classes only. If the image has been graded as 0 by the medical expert, then it is considered as "Normal," if the image has been classified into anything from 1 to 4, then it is considered "Abnormal."

7.2.2 Augmentation of Dataset

The medical datasets that are present in the public domain have less images since the classifier trained on these datasets may get overfitted. This drawback is removed by performing augmentation of dataset using different techniques which enhances the dataset. Augmentation methods are applied to the training part of the dataset, and for every image six augmented images are obtained. Histogram equalization is applied to generate the first image and it helps in enhancing the image contrast. Horizontal flip and vertical flip are used to obtain the next two images. When a mirror image is generated along Y-axis passing through image's mid-point, then the horizontal flip image is generated. Correspondingly, when a mirror image is generated along the X-axis passing through the image's mid-point, the vertical flip image is obtained. The image is counter-clockwise rotated by 90°, 180°, and 270°, respectively to obtain the rest of the images.

7.2.3 Partition of Dataset

As already mentioned, the IDRID dataset is already partitioned into training and testing parts. Therefore, training set is not changed and it contains 413 images. On these images, data augmentation is thereafter executed and the total images on which the networks are trained is equal to 2478. However, testing set is divided into two parts. One part is used for validation and contains 52 images, while the other part is used for testing and it contains 51 images. The validation part is applied for obtaining the appropriate values of hyper-parameters. Lastly, the testing part is used to determine the actual correctness of the architecture.

7.2.4 Evaluation Metrics

The subsequent metrics are used to compute the classification results.

1. **Accuracy:** Accuracy is obtained by placing the number of accurate predictions in the numerator and total number of predictions in the denominator:

$$Accuracy = \frac{TP + TN}{TP + TN + FP + FN}$$

   where, TP stands for true positive and it shows the number of images that are classified correctly to be having diabetic retinopathy. Correspondingly, TN stands for true negative and it denotes the number of images classified correctly as DR negative; i.e., normal. FP stands for false positive and it shows the number of normal images that are wrongly classified as abnormal. Lastly, FN stands for false positive and it denotes abnormal images classified wrongly as normal images.
2. **Area under the curve (AUC):** To obtain the ROC curve, the true positive rate (TPR) and the false positive rate (FPR) is plotted at different threshold values. ROC curve is used to demonstrate the ability of a classifier to diagnose the disease as the threshold value is modified. On the other hand, AUC helps in computing the region or the area enclosed by the ROC curve. AUC is used to describe the probability of a pair, which is random case having one positive and one negative case, being classified correctly.

7.2.5 Method

The method consists of three architectures which include GoogleNet, ResNet and AlexNet. The architectures are modified to perform diabetic retinopathy classification and then from the beginning they are trained. The values of hyper-parameters for all these architectures are separately altered to provide maximum performance. The following is the brief description of these architectures.

AlexNet: This is a long CNN networkproposed by Krizhevsky et al. [19] to perform categorization of images into different classes. It triggered the evolution of many new deep architectures. AlexNet comprises of eight decisive layers, which comprise five convolutional layers followed by three FC (fully-connected) layers. Each convolutional layer has a max-pooling layer placed subsequently. The initial two convolutional layers have a local contrast normalization (LRN) layer placed between the convolutional and max-pooling layer. ReLU stands for Rectified Linear Unit and is used as an activation descriptor in all the convolutional layers. Different sized filters are incorporated by different convolutional layers in the network. The original network was executed on two GPUs; however, it can be executed on one GPU as well. The layerwise architectural detail of AlexNet is depicted in Figure 7.1 and Table 7.1. For more details, refer to Krizhevsky paper [19].

Optimized values of Hyper-parameters: AlexNet is modified to work on fundus images. Here, images of 227×227×1 size are used as input and modified FC layer is used so that it gives only two output values. To optimize the hyper-parameters, manual

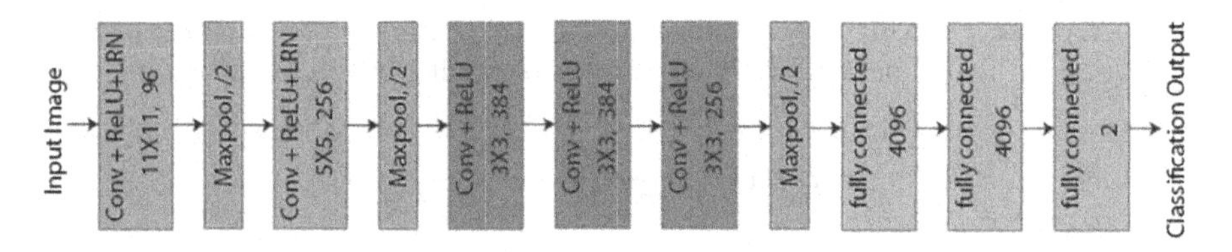

FIGURE 7.1 AlexNet Architecture.

TABLE 7.1
Details of AlexNet Architecture

Layers	# of Filters	Filter Size	Stride	Output Size
Conv +ReLU	96	11×11	4	55×55×96
Maxpool	–	3×3	2	27×27×96
LRN	–	–	–	27×27×96
Conv +ReLU	256	5×5	1	27×27×256
Maxpool	–	3×3	2	13×13×256
LRN	–	–	–	13×13×256
Conv +ReLU	384	3×3	1	13×13×384
Conv +ReLU	384	3×3	1	13×13×384
Conv +ReLU	256	3×3	1	13×13×256
Maxpool	–	3×3	2	6×6×256
Fully-connected	–	–	–	1×4096
Dropout	Keep probability = 0.5			
Fully-connected	–	–	–	1×4096
Dropout	Keep probability = 0.5			
Fully-connected	–	–	–	1×2
Softmax Layer	–	–	–	1

selection is performed. Some of the hyper-parameters are epochs, batch size and learning rate. For weight optimization, training is performed after deciding hyper-parameter values. For optimization, Adam optimization algorithm is used with a starting learning rate of 5×10^{-3}. This learning is decayed at 4% rate after each 300 steps. Batch size used in the training process is 80 images. Batch size is used because large networks have a huge number of parameters and thus all training images cannot be given at one time. The architecture is run 180 times or epochs and each run has 31 steps. This means that architecture is trained for a total of 5580 steps. Network training is begun with random weights and constant biases.

GoogleNet: It is a classification network that was developed by Szegedy et al. [20] in 2014. The network has 22 layers and the USP of the network is the origination of the inception layers. In the initial part, the network uses convolution and max-pooling operations, and thereafter nine inception layers are applied one after another. In every inception layer, the input is parallelly convolved by applying different sized filters. These different sized filters help in improving the scaling invariance of the network. However, it also explodes the number of parameters which is a bottleneck for the execution of the network. This bottleneck is removed by using 1×1 convolutions before higher sized convolutional layers. These 1×1 convolutions help in dimensionality reduction and thus reduce the parameters of the network comprehensively. The layer information of the network is presented in Figure 7.2.

Optimized values of Hyper-parameters: Here, images of 224×224×1 size are used as input and modified FC layer is used so that it gives only two output values after which softmax layer is used for classification. For optimization, Gradient descent optimization algorithm is used with a starting learning rate of 10^{-3}. This learning is decayed at 4% rate after each 4000 steps. Batch size used in the training process is 16 images. The architecture is run for 60 times or epochs and each run has 155 steps. This means that architecture is trained for total of 9300 steps. Network training is begun with using Xavier initializer for weights and constant biases.

ResNet: This network is developed by He et al. [21] and it stands for *residual networks.* The network has different variations and in this study, ResNet-34 is used that has 34 layers. In ResNet, the skip layers are used in which the output of some

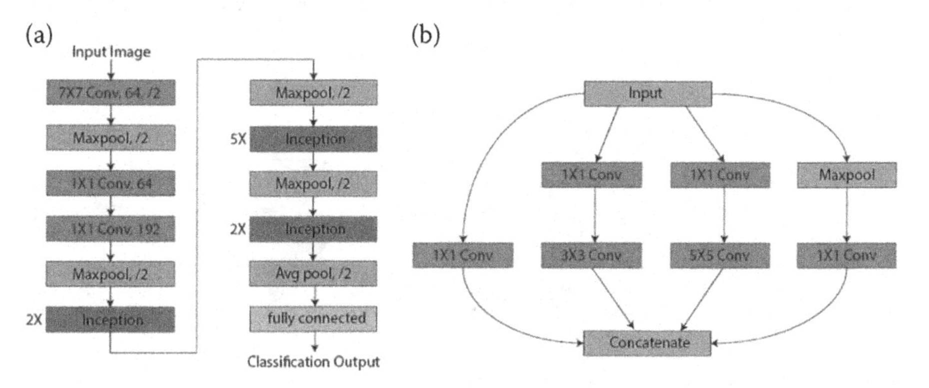

FIGURE 7.2 (a) GoogleNet Network (b) Inception Module.

layers are skipped and is given as input to a layer that is placed later in the network. The architecture consists of 33 convolutional layers and one FC layer. After every two convolutional layers, a skip connection is used, as shown in Figure 7.3. The architecture is used because it converges faster and provides better performance than other deep architectures.

Optimized values of Hyper-parameters: Here, images of 224×224×1 size are used as input and modified FC layer is used so that it gives only two output values after which softmax layer is used for classification. For optimization, Gradient descent optimization algorithm is used with a starting learning rate of 10^{-3}. This learning is decayed at 0.96 rate after each 230 steps. Mini-batch size used in the training process is 128 images. The architecture is run for 30 times or epochs and each run has 20 steps. This means that architecture is trained for a total 600 steps. Network training is begun using random weights and constant biases.

After computing the performance of these three standard networks, an ensemble is built using them. Ensemble is obtained by combining different deep networks by using some blending method. In this study, various ensembles are generated and tested by taking contrasting weights for each separate network. Here, validation set is also applied to find the best weights for each network and these weights are enforced on testing set to realize the eventual performance of the ensemble. The final weights are obtained by varying the weights from 0 to 1 with an increment value of 0.1. This produced various different settings which are tested to obtained the final weights for each architecture. In this study, 0.3, 0.1 and 0.6 weights respectively for Alexnet, GoogleNet and ResNet are used to develop the best performing ensemble.

7.3 RESULTS

In Figures 7.4 and 7.5, the training performance of the individual networks are shown. Each network is trained for different amounts of time by applying distinct hyper-parameters as discussed in Section 3. The training performance shown here verifies that the networks are converged and training is done properly.

During training, validation accuracy is evaluated after each epoch using the set of validation images. This metric is used for the tuning of hyper-parameters and

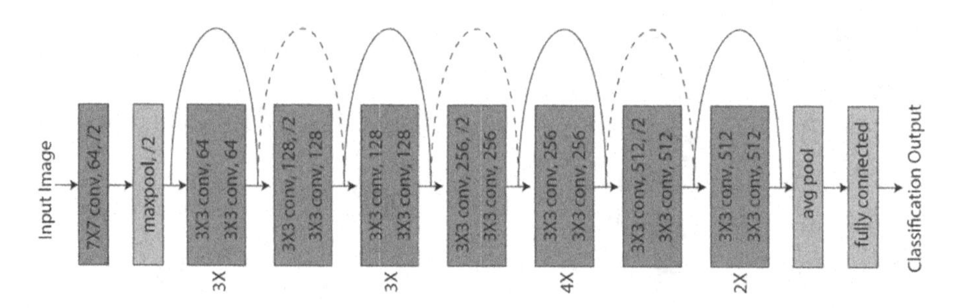

FIGURE 7.3 ResNet Network.

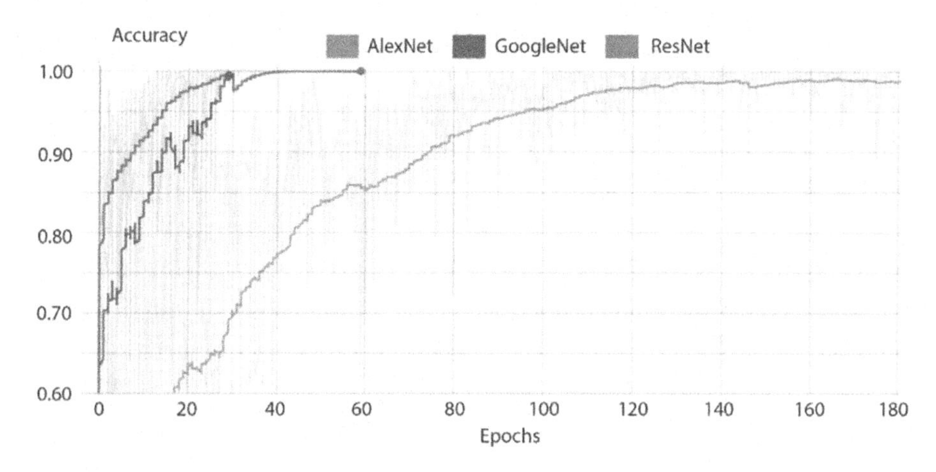

FIGURE 7.4 Training Accuracy of Different Architectures.

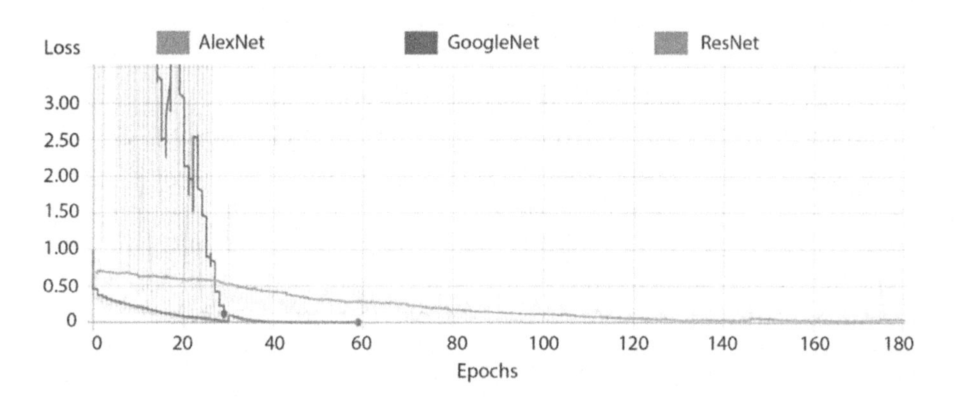

FIGURE 7.5 Training Loss of Different Architectures.

further analyzing the performance of the network on new images using testing set. The final performances of all networks are evaluated on the same testing set. The three standard networks are used to develop an ensemble based on the weighted sum assigned to each architecture. The performance of ensemble and the three networks is shown in Table 7.1. ROC curves of various networks are compared and plotted in Figure 7.6. The classifier with ROC curve having higher AUC is considered more accurate as compared to others. Generally, a classifier having AUC larger than 0.9 is considered a great performer. It can be said by analyzing different computation metrics that the presented ensemble method works better than individual networks by analyzing individual networks.

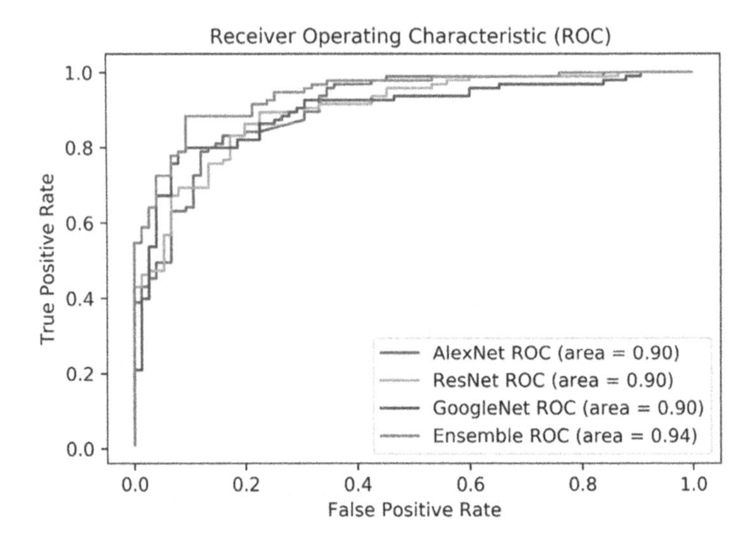

FIGURE 7.6 ROC Curve of Different Architectures.

TABLE 7.2
Computed Accuracy and AUC of Various Networks

Architecture	Accuracy	Area under the Curve (AUC)
AlexNet [18]	82.35	0.90
GoogleNet [19]	80.39	0.90
ResNet [20]	84.31	0.90
Ensemble	88.23	0.94

7.4 CONCLUSION

In this paper, an ensemble has been presented to classify the colored images into Normal and DR class. The ensemble achieved the accuracy of 88.23% which is better than each of the standard architecture that has been used in this study. The ensemble can be used in Primary Health Centers (PHCs) to detect cases that have high probability of having diabetic retinopathy and thus refer these cases to expert doctors. The study can further be extended by classifying the retinal images into different classes based on the severity of the disease.

REFERENCES

1. NCD Risk Factor Collaboration. "Worldwide trends in diabetes since 1980: a pooled analysis of 751 population-based studies with 4·4 million participants." *The Lancet* 387, no. 10027 (2016): 1513–1530.
2. Kapur, Anil, Anthony D. Harries, Knut Lönnroth, Petra Wilson, and Lily SriwahyuniSulistyowati. "Diabetes and tuberculosis co-epidemic: the Bali Declaration." *The Lancet Diabetes & Endocrinology* 4, no. 1 (2016): 8–10.

3. Ege, Bernhard M., Ole K. Hejlesen, Ole V. Larsen, Karina Møller, Barry Jennings, David Kerr, and David A. Cavan. "Screening for diabetic retinopathy using computer based image analysis and statistical classification." *Computer Methods and Programs in Biomedicine* 62, no. 3 (2000): 165–175.
4. Sinthanayothin, Chanjira, Viravud, Kongbunkiat, Suthee, Phoojaruenchanachai, and Apichart Singalavanija. "Automated screening system for diabetic retinopathy." In *3rd International Symposium on Image and Signal Processing and Analysis, 2003. ISPA 2003. Proceedings of the*, vol. 2, pp. 915–920. IEEE, 2003.
5. Vallabha, Deepika, Ramprasath, Dorairaj, Kamesh Namuduri, and Hilary Thompson. "Automated detection and classification of vascular abnormalities in diabetic retinopathy." In *Conference Record of the Thirty-Eighth Asilomar Conference on Signals, Systems and Computers, 2004.*, vol. 2, pp. 1625–1629. IEEE, 2004.
6. Sopharak, Akara, Bunyarit, Uyyanonvara, and Sarah Barman. "Automatic exudate detection from non-dilated diabetic retinopathy retinal images using fuzzy c-means clustering." *Sensors* 9, no. 3 (2009): 2148–2161.
7. Gulshan, Varun, Lily Peng, Marc Coram, Martin C. Stumpe, Derek Wu, Arunachalam, Narayanaswamy, Subhashini Venugopalan et al. "Development and validation of a deep learning algorithm for detection of diabetic retinopathy in retinal fundus photographs." *JAMA* 316, no. 22 (2016): 2402–2410.
8. Amin, Javeria, Muhammad Sharif, Mussarat Yasmin, Hussam Ali, and Steven Lawrence Fernandes. "A method for the detection and classification of diabetic retinopathy using structural predictors of bright lesions." *Journal of Computational Science* 19 (2017): 153–164.
9. Li, Xiaogang, Tiantian Pang, Biao Xiong, Weixiang Liu, Ping Liang, and Tianfu Wang. "Convolutional neural networks based transfer learning for diabetic retinopathy fundus image classification." In *2017 10th International Congress on Image and Signal Processing, BioMedical Engineering and Informatics (CISP-BMEI)*, pp. 1–11. IEEE, 2017.
10. Xu, Kele, Dawei Feng, and Haibo Mi. "Deep convolutional neural network-based early automated detection of diabetic retinopathy using fundus image." *Molecules* 22, no. 12 (2017): 2054.
11. Gargeya, Rishab, and Theodore Leng. "Automated identification of diabetic retinopathy using deep learning." *Ophthalmology* 124, no. 7 (2017): 962–969.
12. Akram, M. Usman, Shehzad Khalid, Anam Tariq, Shoab A. Khan, and Farooque Azam. "Detection and classification of retinal lesions for grading of diabetic retinopathy." *Computers in Biology and Medicine* 45 (2014): 161–171.
13. Pratt, Harry, Frans, Coenen, Deborah M. Broadbent, Simon P. Harding, and Yalin Zheng. "Convolutional neural networks for diabetic retinopathy." *Procedia Computer Science* 90 (2016): 200–205.
14. Dutta, Suvajit, Bonthala CS Manideep, Syed MuzamilBasha, Ronnie D. Caytiles, and N. C. S. N. Iyengar. "Classification of diabetic retinopathy images by using deep learning models." *International Journal of Grid and Distributed Computing* 11, no. 1 (2018): 89–106.
15. Wan, Shaohua, Yan Liang, and Yin Zhang. "Deep convolutional neural networks for diabetic retinopathy detection by image classification." *Computers & Electrical Engineering* 72 (2018): 274–282.
16. Zhao, Mengliu, and Ghassan Hamarneh. "Retinal image classification via vasculature-guided sequential attention." In *Proceedings of the IEEE International Conference on Computer Vision Workshops*, 2019.
17. Khan, SharzilHaris, Zeeshan Abbas, and SM Danish Rizvi. "Classification of diabetic retinopathy images based on customised CNN architecture." In *2019 Amity International Conference on Artificial Intelligence (AICAI)*, pp. 244–248. IEEE, 2019.

18. https://biomedicalimaging.org/2018/challenges/
19. Krizhevsky, Alex, Ilya Sutskever, and Geoffrey E. Hinton. "Imagenet classification with deep convolutional neural networks." In *Advances in Neural Information Processing Systems*25 (2012), pp. 1097–1105.
20. Szegedy, C., Liu, W., Jia, Y., Sermanet, P., Reed, S., Anguelov, D., Erhan, D., Vanhoucke, V. and Rabinovich, A.. Going deeper with convolutions. In *Proceedings of the IEEE Conference on Computer Vision and Pattern Recognition*, pp. 1–9, 2015.
21. He, Kaiming, Xiangyu Zhang, Shaoqing Ren, and Jian Sun. "Deep residual learning for image recognition." In *Proceedings of the IEEE Conference on Computer Vision and Pattern Recognition*, pp. 770–778, 2016.

8 Compression of Clinical Images Using Different Wavelet Function

Munish Kumar and Sandeep Kumar

CONTENTS

8.1 INTRODUCTION: BACKGROUND AND NEED OF COMPRESSION

The process of reducing the proportions of pictures without degrading information content in the pictures is called image compression. Pictures size reduction permits most imageries to be kept within a certain volume of drive space. If the image size is reduced without losing the particular information in the image, then the picture is easily and rapidly transmitted to a network with lesser bandwidth and the time required to send the information is also reduced. Reduction is beneficial since it benefits a decrease in the use of exclusive resources, such as storage space or transmit bandwidth [1, 2, 3]. Here are a number of dissimilar ways in which imagery files can be linked.

Health imagery is a method utilized to generate imageries of the human physique for therapeutic purposes or medical science. Medical imaging is often seen as choosing a method which blindly generates pictures of body parts under observation. Measurement and recording methods do not generate pictures but yield information available for display as maps that can be seen as ways to think about medicine [4, 5].

Hospitals need to store all data related to patients. Thus, they need a large amount of space to store that data and broadcast bandwidth to transmit these images over the network. This requires a huge hard disk space. As of 2010, five billion clinical pictures were studied worldwide [4]. There are numerous medical applications; quicker intelligence, perusing enormous quantities of pictures (e.g., volumetric informational collections, picture time arrangement, picture databases) or looking for setting based gritty picture structures and/or quantitative examination of estimated essential information . Any loss of information in medical imaging, while transmitting the picture is intolerable [6, 7]. There is a wide scope of clinical sources, and a significant number of them disregard the little picture subtleties that point to pathology, which can change the conclusion, bringing about genuine human and lawful outcomes. The growing utilization of 3-D descriptions techniques has prompted the search for effective methods for transporting and storing relevant volumetric statistics.

Therefore, it is necessary to compress data (mainly images) so that they take up less space. This is also required to transmit data over the network. There are two kinds of compression techniques: lossless and lossy. Patient data is important so one needs all the information. Therefore, the lossless compression method is used to compress medical images.

Major issues related to medical films:

1. Space is required to store all medical images.
2. High-bandwidth is required for large size images to be transmitted over the network.

These problems can be solved by compression methods. Using these techniques reduces the amount of space required to store medical images and reduces the size of the image. The reduced bandwidth required for a reduced image is low, so more data can be transmitted over a given bandwidth. The speed of transmission also increases. Thus, compression solves these problems [7–12]. In this work, which wavelet is appropriate for a certain clinical picture is determined. The wavelet is a waveform of a successfully finite interval that takes an average rate of zero. Wave states to a situation where this role is called oscillation. Other signal examination techniques can reveal aspects of missing data such as trends, breakpoints, disjointedness in high derivatives, and self-similarity [13, 14, 15, 16]. There are several members in the wavelet family; i.e., Harr, Coiflets, Symlets, Meyer, Biorthogonal and Daubechies and so on [17, 18, 19, 20, 21]. The wavelet-based clinical picture compression and decompression process is shown in Figure 8.1 [11]. Wavelet pressure is a method of examining a compacted picture in a repeatable way, bringing about a progression of high-goals pictures, every one of which 'includes' data substance to low-goals pictures [6, 22].

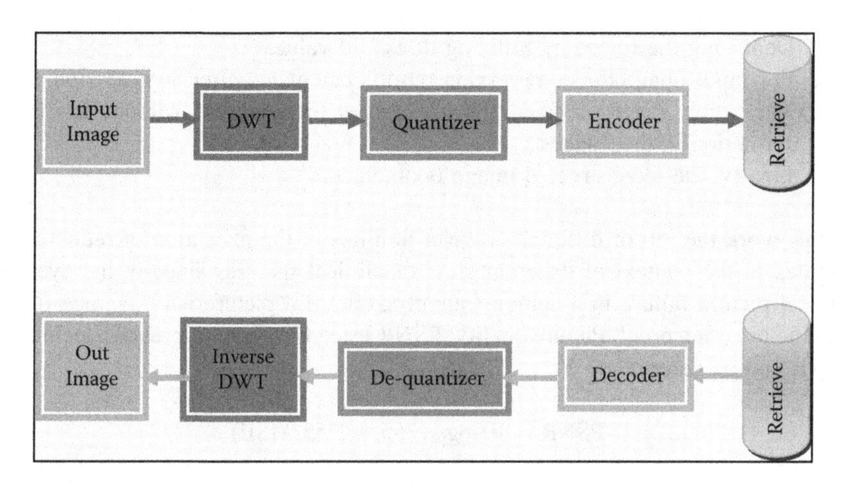

FIGURE 8.1 Clinical Image Compression and Decompression [23].

8.2 TERMINOLOGY UTILIZED FOR IMPLEMENTATION

Various terminologies are utilized in image compression calculations. The value of restored pictures is calculated by comparing the different compression techniques available. Two scientific terms are utilized to measure the value of the restored pictures; namely MSE and PSNR [9]. The PSNR is most regularly utilized as a proportion of nature of reproduction in picture pressure and so forth.

MSE can be characterized as [24]:

$$MSE = \frac{1}{\text{MN}} \sum_{i=0}^{m-1} \sum_{j=0}^{n-1} \| I(i, j) - K(i, j) \| \tag{8.1}$$

and PSNR is given as per:

$$PSNR = 10 \log_{10}\left(\frac{MAX_1^2}{MSE}\right) = 20 \log_{10}\left(\frac{MAX_1}{\sqrt{MSE}}\right) \tag{8.2}$$

In this, I(i, j) - input picture, K(i, j) - approximated adaptation and M, N are the picture components. Low value of MSE and high PSNR value means that compression is better [24].

8.3 PROPOSED ALGORITHM

For compression and decompression of images the basic steps are [22, 25, 26, 27, 28]:

a. Input image is taken from the source/scanner.
b. Image decomposition is performed.
c. Compressed image is created after performing certain steps.

d. Denoising the image by utilizing threshold value.
e. For input image the compression ratio is calculated after compression.
f. The value PSNR is fixed for all images to compress without losing information in the images.
g. Finally, the reconstructed image is obtained.

In this work the job of different wavelet families in the execution of reduction of pictures in the context of different sorts of clinical pictures since in the event of clinical picture failure in a demonstratively zone of a picture isn't average over a specific breaking point. Picture quality, PSNR esteem is fixed of pressure technique. PSNR can be determined as

$$PSNR = 10\log_{10}(255 * 255/MSE) \tag{8.3}$$

PSNR is fixed for each image. Distinctive biomedical pictures with various wavelet families are utilized. Each time an alternate wavelet family is utilized and pressure proportion is determined. Based on that pressure proportion, we propose the most reasonable wavelet work for a given kind of picture.

8.3.1 Calculation for Picture Compression Utilizing Wavelet

So as to choose the most fitting wavelet work for a specific sort of biomedical picture, we utilize the accompanying advances

8.3.1.1 Input Image

First input image is occupied for reduction by utilizing IMREAD ('image') MATLAB command. After that, enter the level of decomposition for image. In this thesis level 2 is used for all images. Figure 8.2 is shown below the input image.

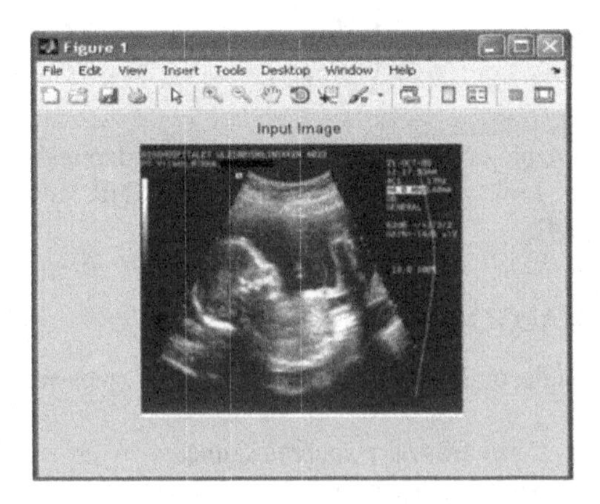

FIGURE 8.2 Input Image.

8.3.1.2 Compression Decompression and Filters

In the subsequent stage ascertain the various channels with sort of function of wavelet.

$$[\text{Lo\_D, Hi\_D, Lo\_R, Hi\_R}] = \text{wfilters}(\text{'wname'}); \tag{8.4}$$

The '4' yield channels are

Lo_D, the decomposition low-pass filter
Hi_D, the decomposition high-pass filter
Lo_R, the reconstruction low-pass filter
Hi_R, the reconstruction high-pass filter

Now perform multilevel decomposition: -

[c, s] = wavedec2 (uint8(X), n, Lo_D, Hi_D);

Formation of vector C as follow: -

$$\begin{aligned} C = [&A(N)|H(N)|V(N)|D(N)|\ldots H(N-1)|V(N-1)| \\ &D(N-1)\ldots H(1)|V(1)|D(1)]. \end{aligned} \tag{8.5}$$

In this A - approximation coefficients, H - horizontal details, V - vertical details, D - diagonal details. Figure 8.3 show the network of vector; every vector is the vector segment savvy stockpiling of a lattice. Grid S is with the end goal.

$$\begin{aligned} &S(1, :) = \text{estimation coefficients size}(N) \\ &S(i, :) = \text{detail coefficients size}(N - i + 2) \\ &\text{for } I = 2, \ldots N + 1 \text{ and } S(N + 2, :) = \text{size}(X). \end{aligned} \tag{8.6}$$

Close to this default an incentive for the compression.

$$[\text{THR, SORH, KEEPAPP, CRIT}] = \text{DDENCMP}(\text{'cmp', 'wp', uint8(X)}); \tag{8.7}$$

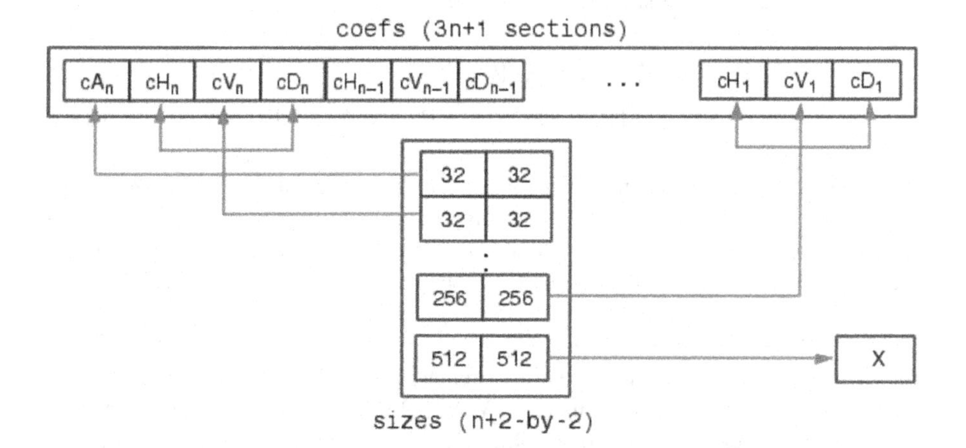

FIGURE 8.3 Matrix of Vectors.

8.3.1.3 Compression

By using wavelet function compression is performed on output image from previous steps.

$$[XC, TREED, PERF0, PERFL2] = WPDENCMP(X, SORH, 2, \text{'wname'}, CRIT, THR, KEEPAPP); \quad (8.8)$$

By using MATLAB function compression or de-noising is performed on the details or images.

$$[XD, TREED, PERF0, PERFL2] = \text{wpdencmp}(X, SORH, N, \text{'wname'}, CRIT, PAR, KEEPAPP). \quad (8.9)$$

Restores de-noise or compacted adaptation XD information sign X got through wavelet bundles coefficients thresholding.

PERFL2 and PERF0 are L2 vitality restoration and compressor levels in rates.

$$PERFL2 = 100 * (\text{vector-standard of WP-cfs of XD/vector-standard of WP-cfs of X})2 \quad (8.10)$$

On the off chance that X is a 1-D symbol and 'name' a symmetrical wavelet, PERFL2 is diminished to

$$SORH(\text{'s' or' h'}) \text{where 's'- soft, h- hard thresholding} \quad (8.11)$$

For better decomposition entropy method is used by string CRIT and PAR parameter. PAR is like thresholding. In the event that KEEPAPP = 1, estimation coefficients can't be thresholder; else, can be.

$$[XD, TREED, PERF0, PERFL2] = \text{wpdencmp}(TREE, SORH, CRIT, PAR, KEEPAPP) \quad (8.12)$$

have a similar yield contention, utilizing indistinguishable alternatives from above, yet got legitimately from the info wavelet type decomposition 'TREE' of sign to be de-noised or packed. What's more if CRIT = 'nobest' no improvement is done and the present disintegration is limited. The original image and the output image are shown in Figure 8.4.

8.3.1.4 Image Reconstruction

In this progression staggered 2-D wavelet remaking of 'n' level of deterioration happens out = waverec2(c, s, 'wname'); WAVEREC2 plays out a staggered two-dimensional wavelet reconstructing utilizing either a particular wavelet ('wname') or

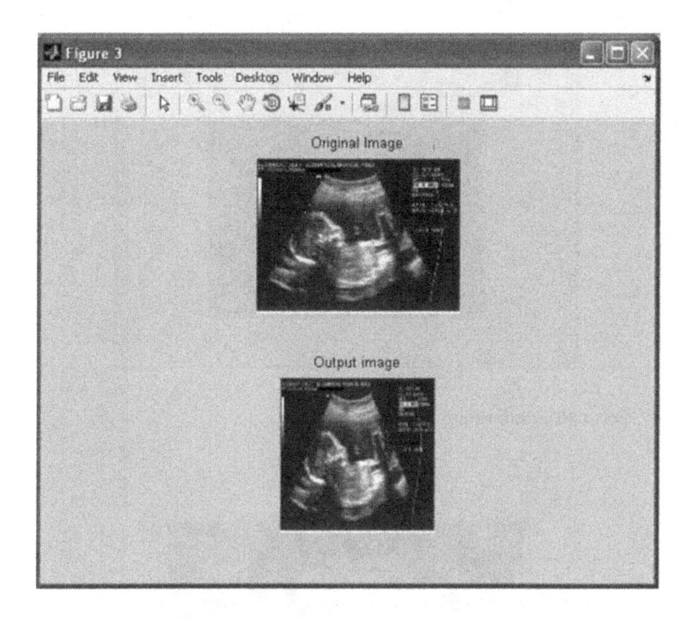

FIGURE 8.4 Original and Output Image.

explicit reproduction channels (Lo_R and Hi_R). X = WAVEREC2(C, S, 'wname') remakes framework 'X' dependent upon staggered wavelet decay structure [C, S].

$$\text{For } X = \text{WAVEREC2}(C, S, Lo\_R, Hi\_R), \tag{8.13}$$

where Lo_R- low-pass filter & Hi_R- high-pass filter

n-level reconstructed picture is shown in Figure 8.5.

8.3.2 Performance Analysis

In the above calculation the valve of PSNR is fixed for a given kind of picture. Now we determined the reduction proportion at last advance as PERFO shows the data compression approval. As the PSNR esteem is fixed one can examine the pressure proportion of a specific clinical picture with each sort of wavelet work and can choose which wavelet is generally appropriate for that specific kind of clinical picture. Figure 8.6 shows the yield picture.

These means have been performed for pressure by utilizing distinctive sorts of wavelet capacity to a given kind of clinical picture and to recommend the most proper wavelet work that can perform ideal pressure for that picture.

8.4 IMPLEMENTATION AND RESULT

Image size reduction is performed by utilizing wavelets and computing the compression proportion by means of various wavelet types. The consequences of the

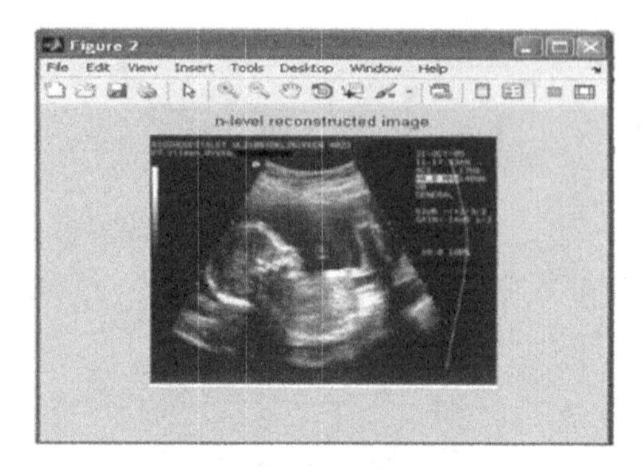

FIGURE 8.5 Reconstructed Image.

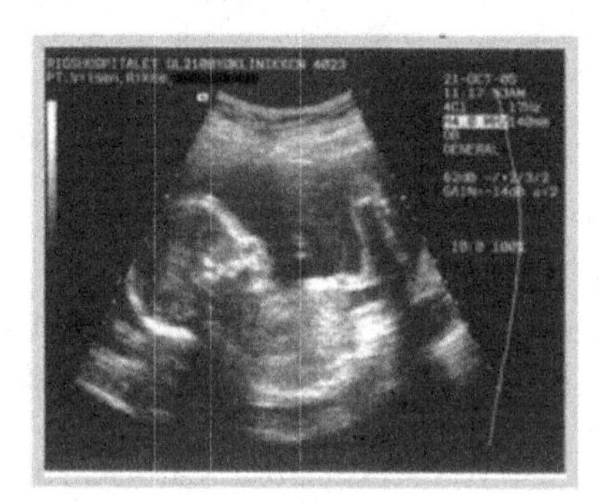

FIGURE 8.6 Final Yield Picture.

pressure proportion for various types of wavelets are shown in table. The wavelet type which gives greatest compression without loss of information for a specific sort of clinical picture would be the most proper wavelet for that kind of clinical picture. Limit and PSNR are set with the goal that their qualities are consistently reliable for a given sort of picture pressure. Continue rehashing this pressure for an alternate sort of wavelet works and ascertain the pressure proportion that can be accomplished with every one of them. The following is the yield of each sort of picture pressure with various wavelet capacities.

8.4.1 Analysis of CT Scan Images

The CT scan imageries would be analyzing for dissimilar wavelet changes.

8.4.1.1 Wavelet Haar Function Is Used

First input image is taken after that modifies those pictures in 256*256 dimensions; i.e., 256 no. of rows and 256 no. of columns for input image.

Step I: Decomposition Vector Level Is Set

In this 'n' level decomposition used for the sample pictures is engaged, in which the value of 'n' is set to 2. After that calculate the different filters associated with certain kind of wavelet occupation and perform multilevel decomposition. Figure 8.7 shows input image.

Here is situated an exact edge level, on the basis that the unique pictures are recovered and n-level compressed imageries where the rebuilding is through giving to HAAR technique. Figure 8.8 shows a reconstructed image of CT scan using HAAR wavelet.

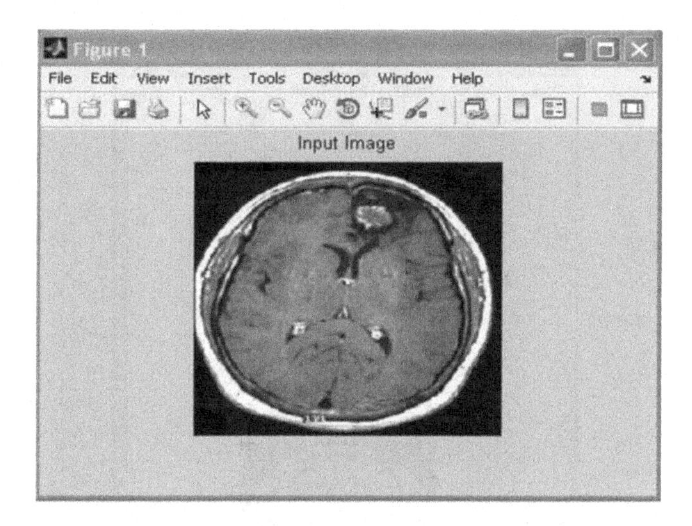

FIGURE 8.7 CT Scan Input Image.

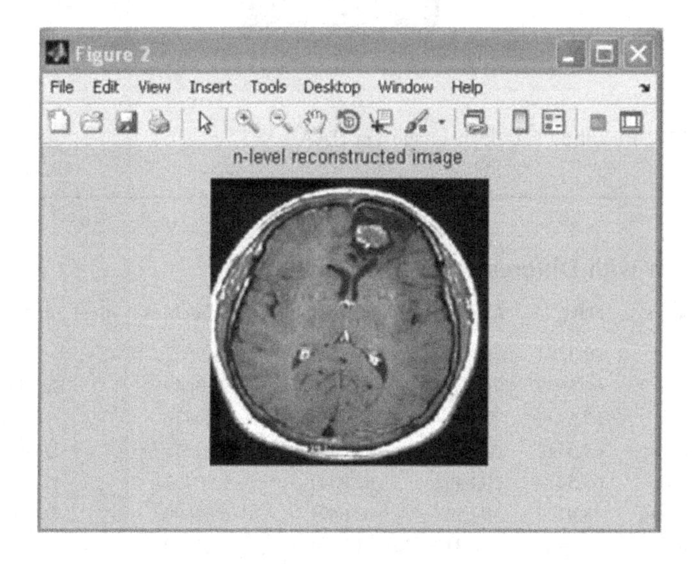

FIGURE 8.8 Reconstructed Image of CT Scan via HAAR WT.

Step 2: Resulting Pictures

In Figure 8.9, the PSNR is 7.7246 after two stage reconstructed image. The ratio of compression is 59.8679% attend. In a similar manner for all the images these operations are performed and calculations made. From Table 8.1 the conclusion is made that the pressure proportion is obtained after every pressure and the wavelet capacity chosen that can provide the greatest pressure proportion to a specific clinical picture. In this examination distinctive wavelet capacities are applied on various sorts of clinical pictures for a fix PSNR esteem and the pressure proportion is determined. Figure 8.10 illustrates the outcome of the analysis of various medical images.

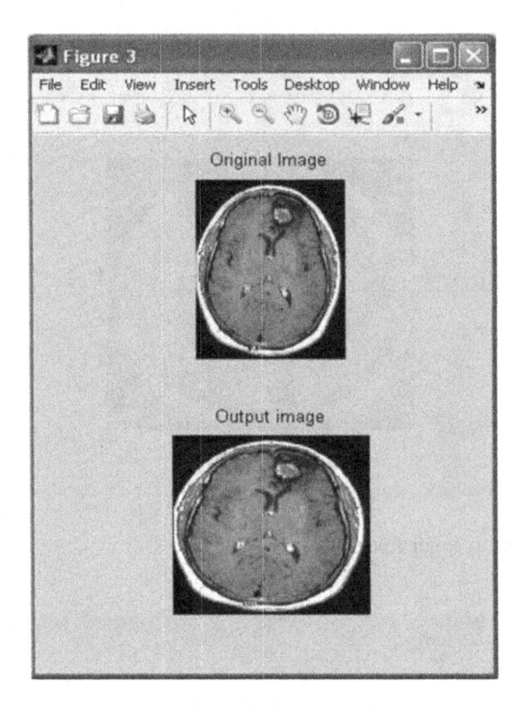

FIGURE 8.9 Resulting CT Scan Image via HAAR WT.

TABLE 8.1
Result Ratio with Different Wavelet Families

Clinical Images	Harr	Coiflets	Biorthogonal	Daubechies	Best Suitable Wavelet
X-ray	79.3284	82.4315	81.8641	81.9552	Coiflets
CT images	59.8679	70.2613	74.9806	71.9649	Biorthogonal
MRI images	69.6737	77.8837	77.3635	76.0476	Coiflets
Ultrasound	64.5142	64.8895	66.4457	67.2255	Daubechies
Mammography	60.5475	67.8532	67.8947	72.0437	Daubechies
Optical imaging	48.9726	59.6248	60.6491	65.4690	Daubechies
Maximum value	79.3284	82.4315	81.8641	81.9552	

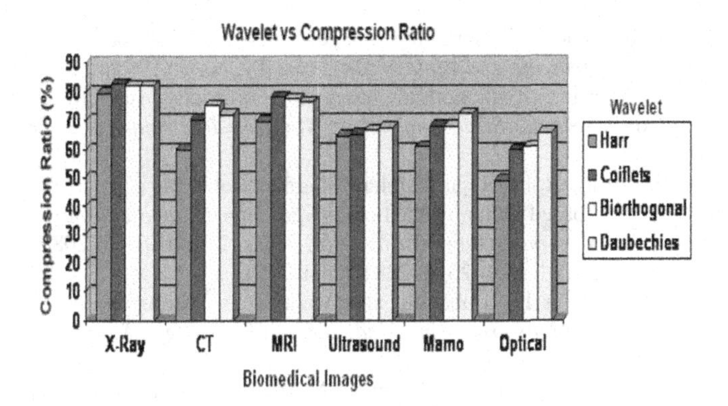

FIGURE 8.10 Wavelet vs Compression Ratio.

8.5 CONCLUSION

In this paper, various types of wavelets are applied to dissimilar types of medical pictures with constant value of PSNR and compression ratio is calculated as a percentage. Since hospitals need to store all data related to patients, they need a large amount of space to store that data. Transmission requires large bandwidth when transmitting data over the network. Compression is necessary to solve these problems. If we want to upload medical images on the Internet, we have to compress the images. Compression images can be easily uploaded and easily downloaded. Also, we can share images on low bandwidth over the network.

After the analysis findings, the coefficients for the X-ray pictures can give the finest outcome as the compression ratio is 82.4315%. Biorthogonal image for CT scan images gives the finest outcome as its compression ratio is 74.9806. The Coiflets image for MRI images gives good outcomes compared to other wavelet roles because it provides a compression ratio of almost 77.8837%. For the ultrasound pictures, the Daubcheese model gives a good outcome and ratio of compression is 67.2255%. For the mammography pictures, Daubcheese model performs a high ratio of compression up to 72.0437%. For optical images 'Daubechies' make available the good outcome and its compression ratio is 65.4690%. This result is the result of the analysis of various medical pictures. In this examination, the threshold and PSNR value for each picture is determined and uses dissimilar wavelets to compress each picture. The compression ratio is analyzed in percentage attained after each compression and determines whether a wavelet job can make available the all-out compression ratio for a specific clinical picture.

REFERENCES

1. Richardson, Walter B., "Applying wavelets to mammograms," *IEEE Engineering in Medicine and Biology Magazine* 14, no. 5 (1995): 551–560.
2. Yang, Zeshang, Maria Kallergi, Ronald A. DeVore, Bradley J. Lucier, Wei Qian, Robert A. Clark, and Laurence P. Clarke. "Effect of wavelet bases on compressing digital mammograms." *IEEE Engineering in Medicine and Biology Magazine* 14, no. 5 (1995): 570–577.

3. Manduca, Armando. "Compressing images with wavelet/subband coding." *IEEE Engineering in Medicine and Biology Magazine* 14, no. 5 (1995): 639–646.
4. Daubechies, Ingrid. "Orthonormal bases of compactly supported wavelets II. Variations on a theme." *SIAM Journal on Mathematical Analysis* 24, no. 2 (1993): 499–519.
5. Laxmikant Tiwari, Rohit Raja, Vaibhav Sharma, Rohit Miri, Adaptive neuro fuzzy inference system based fusion of medical image, *International Journal of Research in Electronics and Computer Engineering*, Vol. 7, Iss. 2, (2019) pp. 2086–2091, ISSN: 2393–9028 (PRINT) |ISSN: 2348–2281 (ONLINE).
6. Kjoelen, Arve, Scott E. Umbaugh, and Mark Zuke. "Compression of skin tumor images." *IEEE Engineering in Medicine and Biology Magazine* 17, no. 3 (1998): 73–80.
7. Zeng, Li, Christian P. Jansen, Stephan Marsch, Michael Unser, and Patrick R. Hunziker. "Four-dimensional wavelet compression of arbitrarily sized echocardiographic data." *IEEE Transactions on Medical Imaging* 21, no. 9 (2002): 1179–1187.
8. Buccigrossi, Robert W., and Eero P. Simoncelli. "Image compression via joint statistical characterization in the wavelet domain." *IEEE Transactions on Image Processing* 8, no. 12 (1999): 1688–1701.
9. Nikita Rawat, Rohit Raja. Moving vehicle detection and tracking using modified mean shift method and Kalman filter and research, *International Journal of New Technology and Research (IJNTR)*, Vol. 2, Iss. 5, (2016): pp. 96–100, ISSN: 2454–4116.
10. Nagaria, Baluram, MHD Farukh Hashmi, and Pradeep Dhakad. "Comparative analysis of fast wavelet transform for image compression for optimal image quality and higher compression ratio." *International Journal of Engineering Science and Technology* 3, no. 5 (2011) pp. 4014–4019.
11. Badawy, Wael, Michael Weeks, Guoqing Zhang, Michael Talley, and Magdy A. Bayoumi. "MRI data compression using a 3-D discrete wavelet transform." *IEEE Engineering in Medicine and Biology Magazine* 21, no. 4 (2002): 95–103.
12. Xiong, Zixiang, Xiaolin Wu, Samuel Cheng, and Jianping Hua. "Lossy-to-lossless compression of medical volumetric data using three-dimensional integer wavelet transforms." *IEEE Transactions on Medical Imaging* 22, no. 3 (2003): 459–470.
13. Graps, Amara. "An introduction to wavelets." *IEEE Computational Science and Engineering* 2, no. 2 (1995): 50–61.
14. Grgic, Mislav, Mario Ravnjak, and Branka Zovko-Cihlar. "Filter comparison in wavelet transform of still images." In ISIE'99. Proceedings of the IEEE International Symposium on Industrial Electronics (Cat. No. 99TH8465), vol. 1, pp. 105–110. IEEE, 1999.
15. Li, Xiaojuan, Guangshu Hu, and Shangkai Gao. "Design and implementation of a novel compression method in a tele-ultrasound system." *IEEE Transactions on Information Technology in Biomedicine* 3, no. 3 (1999): 205–213.
16. Shapiro, Jerome M. "Embedded image coding using zerotrees of wavelet coefficients." *IEEE Transactions on Signal Processing* 41, no. 12 (1993): 3445–3462.
17. Daubechies, Ingrid. "Orthonormal bases of compactly supported wavelets." *Communications on Pure and Applied Mathematics* 41, no. 7 (1988): 909–996.
18. Menegaz, Gloria, and J-P. Thiran. "Three-dimensional encoding/two-dimensional decoding of medical data." *IEEE Transactions on Medical Imaging* 22, no. 3 (2003): 424–440.
19. Rohit Raja, Tilendra Shishir Sinha, Ravi Prakash Dubey. Recognition of human-face from side-view using progressive switching pattern and soft-computing technique, Association for the Advancement of Modelling and Simulation Techniques in Enterprises, Advance B, 58, N 1, (2015): pp. 14–34, ISSN: 1240–4543.

20. Dilmaghani, Reza Sham, A. Ahmadian, Mohammad Ghavami, and A. Hamid Aghvami. "Progressive medical image transmission and compression." *IEEE Signal Processing Letters* 11, no. 10 (2004): 806–809.
21. Chiu, Ed, Jacques Vaisey, and M. Stella Atkins. "Wavelet-based space-frequency compression of ultrasound images." *IEEE Transactions on Information Technology in Biomedicine* 5, no. 4 (2001): 300–310.
22. Munish Kumar and Priyanka, "Medical image compression using different wavelet families", *International Journal of Engineering, Science and Metallurgy* 2, no. 3 (2012), pp 681–684.
23. Rohit Raja, Tilendra Shishir Sinha, Raj Kumar Patra and Shrikant Tiwari. Physiological trait based biometrical authentication of human-face using LGXP and ANN techniques, *International Journal of Information and Computer Security* 10, nos. 2/3 (2018): pp. 303–320.
24. Zettler, William R., John C. Huffman, and David CP Linden. "Application of compactly supported wavelets to image compression." In Image processing algorithms and techniques 1244, pp. 150–160. International Society for Optics and Photonics, 1990.
25. Sudeepti Neelesh, Gupta and Sharma, Neetu "Image Compression on Region of Interest based on SPIHT Algorithm" *International Journal of Computer Applications* (0975–8887), 132, no. 11 (2015), pp. 41–45.
26. Kumar S. and Munish Kumar, "A review on image compression technique" in International Conference PPIMT Hisar and Paper ID: SBT-125.
27. Kumar S, Sanjay Sharma, and Sandeep Singh, "Image compression based on ISPIHT and region of interest and hardware implementations" in International Conference OITM Hisar and Paper ID: RTCMC-209.
28. Kumar S., Munish Kumar, and Kapil Gulati, "An overview of mammography" in AICTE sponsored National Conference on (ETEC-2013) held on October 25–26 in collaboration with International Journal of Computer Application at BRCMCET, Bahal.

9 PSO-Based Optimized Machine Learning Algorithms for the Prediction of Alzheimer's Disease

Saroj Kumar Pandey, Rekh Ram Janghel, Pankaj Kumar Mishra, Kshitiz Varma, Prashant Kumar, and Saurabh Dewangan

CONTENTS

9.1 INTRODUCTION

Until now Support Vector Machine (SVM) has been successfully applied for solving data classification and regression problems as it is a Supervised Learning algorithm and gives outstanding performance and computation cost [1]. It should be mentioned that in SVM implementation the classification performance of SVM is largely dependent on the random parameter selection. If it is not chosen properly 'it may cause poor robustness of the classifier'. In order to improve the performance or effectiveness of Support Vector Machine, a natural idea is to use Evolutionary computation

(EC) algorithms for optimizing 'the parameters of 'Support Vector Machine.' In search of a suitable EC algorithm, the Particle Swarm Optimization (PSO) approach proposed by Kennedy and Eberhart [2] appears to be one of the best options available'. 'PSO is a population-based stochastic optimization algorithm which follow 'the behavior of organisms such as birds flocking and fishing schooling'. In this study, we have used machine learning algorithms such as Support Vector Machine Classification, Random Forest Classification, XgBoost Classifier, Decision Tree Classification, Adaboost Classifier, K-Neighbour Classifier and Logistic Regression, along with Particle Swarm Optimization technique in order to classify Alzheimer's Disease. Classification is one of the important things so that we are able to distinguish whether the person is suffering from Alzheimer's Disease or not. Classification of 'Alzheimer's disease has been always challenging and most problematic part has been always selecting the most discriminative features'.

Alzheimer's Disease is a kind of neurodegenerative disease of the central nervous system characterized by progressive cognitive impairment. 'Sixth main cause of death with a rising 'population is Alzheimer's Disease and it is also known as late-life disease. Although there are 'some medical treatment may temporarily show positive effects but 'none has demonstrated the capability of preventing deterioration' [2]. 'Alzheimer's Disease (AD) is the most common type of' disease 'among people 65 years and older. In this disease the mental ability of persons gradually decreases and reaches a stage where it becomes very difficult for them to live a normal life. It is expected that 1 in 85 people will be affected by 2050 and the number of affected people is going to be doubled in the next 20 years [3].

9.2 RELATED WORK

In the field of classification of Alzhiemer's Diseases using machine learning algorithms, these are some previous works. Beheshti et al. [4] proposed a Support Vector Machine based classification machine learning algorithm where the main objective is to do Structural MRI-based detection of Alzheimer's disease using feature ranking and classification error. Through this method they have achieved a sensitivity of 80.20%, specificity of 90% and accuracy of 84.90%. Spulber et al. [5] proposed an orthogonal projections to latent structures (OPLS) based classification where the main objective is to do an MRI-based index to measure the severity of Alzheimer's disease-like structural pattern in subjects with mild cognitive impairment; through this means they have achieved a sensitivity of 86.1%, specificity of 90.4% and accuracy of 88.4%. Beheshti et al. [6] proposed a SVM with 10 fold cross-validation based classification machine learning algorithm where the main objective is to do Structural classification of Alzheimer's disease and prediction of mild cognitive impairment-to-Alzheimer's conversion from structural magnetic resource imaging using feature ranking and a genetic algorithm. Through this method, they have achieved a sensitivity of 89.13%, specificity of 96.80% and accuracy of 93.01%. Tong et al. [7] proposed a Random Forest-based classification machine learning algorithm where the main objective is to do a Novel Grading Biomarker for the Prediction of Conversion from Mild Cognitive Impairment to Alzheimer's Disease. Through this method they have achieved a sensitivity of 86.7%, specificity of 72.6% and accuracy of 80.7%. Jayapathy Rajeesh et al. [8] proposed a Support Vector Machine based classification machine learning algorithm where the main objective is to do a Discrimination of Alzheimer's disease using hippocampus texture features from MRI and through this way they have achieved a sensitivity of 91.1%, specificity of 95.9% and accuracy of 93.6%. Zhang et al. [9] proposed a PSO-kernel SVM-DT method where the main objective is to do classification of Alzheimer Disease Based on Structural Magnetic Resonance Imaging by Kernel Support Vector Machine Decision Tree. In this way they have achieved a sensitivity of 98%, specificity of 89% and accuracy of 80%. Shih-Ting Yang et al. [10] proposed a PSO-SVM method where the main objective is to do Discrimination between Alzheimer's Disease and Mild Cognitive Impairment Using SOM and PSO-SVM. Through this method, they have achieved a sensitivity of 94.12%, specificity of 94.12% and accuracy of 94.12%. M. Evanchalin Sweety et al. [11] proposed a PSO – Decision Tree method where the main objective is to do Detection of Alzheimer Disease in Brain Images Using PSO and Decision Tree Approach. Through this method they have achieved a sensitivity of 88.10%, specificity of 85.16% and accuracy of 86.89%. Wang et al. [12] proposed a PSO-Kernal SVM method where the main objective is to do an MR Brain Images Classifier System via Particle Swarm Optimization and Kernel Support Vector Machine. Through this method, they achieved a sensitivity of 98.12%, specificity of 92% and accuracy of 97.78%. Sivapriya et al. [13] proposed a PSO-LSSVM method where the main objective is to do Automated Classification of Dementia Using PSO based Least Square Support Vector Machine. Through this means they have achieved a sensitivity of 95%, specificity of 97% and accuracy of 96%.

9.3 MATERIAL AND METHODS

9.3.1 Proposed Workflow

In the proposed workflow, we are starting from ADNI (Alzheimer's disease Neuroimaging Initiative) which is a website that provides the dataset of Alzheimer's disease. After obtaining the dataset we are preprocessing so that in future when we apply some machine learning algorithms will get some good results. After preprocessing the data, we divide the data set into two sets, first is training

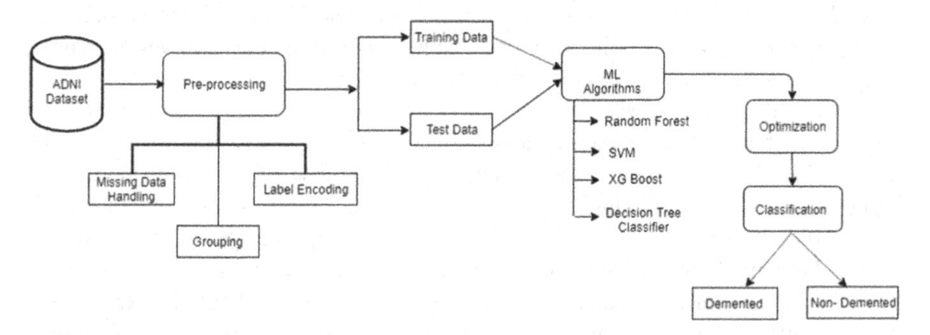

FIGURE 9.1 Workflow Diagram of Proposed Method of Alzheimer's Classification.

data set with which we train our model and second is test dataset with which we can be sure that our model is trained properly and it is giving good results. After dividing dataset we pick up seven machine learning algorithms that we have defined earlier to train these ML model;s and for obtaining better accuracy we use Particle Swarm Optimization technique; finally, after applying optimization we can classify people as either demented or non-demented.

9.3.2 Database

The dataset that are used in this paper was taken from the (ADNI) database which stands Alzheimer's Disease Neuroimaging Initiative, 'which was launched in 2003 by''the National Institute on Aging (NIA)', the Food and Drug Administration (FDA)', 'and the National Institute of Biomedical Imaging and Bioengineering (NIBIB) '[2].' 'We' split the dataset 'into two' sets; i.e., 'training'data and 'testing'data. In this study, we acquired data from Alzheimer's Disease Neurological Initiative (ADNI). The dataset that we have used is in CSV format and it is converted form of Image ADNI dataset.

9.3.3 Data Pre-processing

For pre-processing of data, we have done the following:

- Missing Data Handling
- Grouping
- Label Encoding

Missing Data Handling: Data collected from soe sources has some type of inconsistency, either due to redundancy or because some data could be missing from the columns and rows. This needs to be addressed so that calculations done by a machine learning algorithm can provide better results. Handling missing data from the dataset could be more challenging because it requires some analytics done in such a way that the data which we are going to put into the place should help us in better implementation of algorithms. Let us look at different ways of imputing the missing values [14]. There are null values which need to be handled. The Delete Row method is used for it. In this, we can follow two courses. The first one involves deleting a particular row if it has a null value for a feature. The second one involves deleting a particular column if it has 70–75% of its data missing.

We can also apply mode, median and mean strategy on some features. For instance, in the age of a person we can calculate either the mean, the median or the mode values for it and replace the missing cells with those values. Some amount of variance is added in the dataset as a result, but the loss of the same can be negated by incorporating this method which further yields better results. The use of the above three methods for approximation is considered a statistical approach to handle missing values. It is also known as leaking the data while training. One other way is to fill the missing values by approximating the deviation with its neighbors. This method usually works better if the data is linear.

Grouping: Grouping is another preprocessing technique or method which help in differentiating data. According to the values of rows and columns it makes the same type of data and assigns them values according to their effectiveness in the dataset [15].

Label Encoding: With different types of datasets we always come across the kind of data which contains multiple labels in either single or multiple columns. This label can be in the form of words or in the form of numbers Also, to make the human data understandable and to make it more controlled while applying any machine learning algorithm, training data is labelled in words called label encoding. Basically, it is converting the labels into numeric form so that an algorithm can decide in a better way how those labels must be operated. it is one of the important steps for the preprocessing in a supervised learning technique [16].

9.4 PARTICLE SWARM OPTIMIZATION (PSO) TECHNIQUES

Particle swarm optimization (PSO)'is a population-based, 'stochastic, global optimization technique proposed by Kennedy and Eberhart in 1995 [8]'. Particle Swarm Optimization is a unique searching mechanism, with a simple concept, computational efficiency and easy implementation. It is inspired by the social behavior of birds moving together in search of food. Due to this, it has been applied to many optimization areas.

Particle Swarm Optimization algorithm can be outlined as below: We start by giving the swarm a random position in the problem space of each particle.

- For each particle we will calculate fitness function.
- For the particles that are present in swarm we will compare the particle's pbest with its fitness value and if the current value is better than the best value, then we will use this value as the pbest and particle's current position, xi as pi.
- Next, we will identify the particle that has the fitness value best and the value of its fitness function is identified as position as pg and guest.
- If there is a updating in velocity and acceleration, then we will use (1) and (2).
- At last we will perform steps 2–5 until a stopping criterion is met [17].

9.4.1 MACHINE LEARNING MODELS

- Random Forest Classifier
- Support Vector Machine
- Decision Tree Classifier
- XgBoost Classifier
- AdaBoost Classifier
- K- neighbour Classifier
- Logistic Regression

Random Forest Classifier: Random forest is used both for regression and as well as for classification as it is a supervised learning algorithm. With such flexible features, the algorithm can be easily understood. It is like an actual forest comprising trees whose robustness depends upon the number of trees within. On the selected sampled data it randomly creates a decision tree and gets a prediction for each tree. The best solution is selected by voting. For selecting features, it is a good indicator. The application of Random Forest Classifier is in classification of images, selection of features and recommendation engines. It can be used for prediction of disease and in identifying fraud activities. It lies at the base of the Boruta algorithm, which selects important features in a dataset [18, 19].

Support Vector Machine: A Support Vector Machine (SVM) is a classifier that performs discriminative classification that is formally defined by a separating hyper-plane. Basically, the SVM algorithm outputs an optimal hyper-plane that categorizes new examples for labelled training data. This hyper-plane may be a line or curve. For a two-dimensional space it is a line dividing a plane into two parts, wherein each class lay on either side of the plane.

Decision Tree Classifier: A Decision Tree algorithm is a type of supervised learning algorithm. This algorithm can be used for both regression and classification. It learns to predict target variables by forming different decision trees using previously known data or information. It uses tree representation to solve the problem, which is fairly simple and easy to understand. All the individual nodes represent attributes and all the leaf nodes represent the classes [20, 21, 22].

XgBoost Classifier: Xg-Boost is basically a Decision-tree-based machine learning algorithm and a framework that is used by Xgboost is gradient boosting. Data like images, text, etc. are unstructured problems that are involved in the prediction problem. In the algorithms and framework that are present, Artificial Neural Networks tend to outperform. However, decision tree-based algorithms are considered the best in class algorithm when it is a matter of small-medium structured/tabular data.

Ada-boost Classifier: Ada-boost is another ensemble classifier like random forest classifier. (The combination of multiple classification algorithms is known as ensemble classifier and output is calculated by using a combined result of the output of those algorithms.) In this area, we mainly describe the database and proposed methodology.

9.5 EXPERIMENTAL RESULTS

System Configuration: Our system configuration consists of HP and Lenovo laptops with the configuration of 8GB RAM consisting of Intel core i5 processor. We have used the Jupyter notebook environment for training purposes.

Parameter Evaluation: Table 9.1 consists of seven machine learning algorithms, namely Random Forest, Support Vector Machine, Decision Tree, XgBoost, Adaboost, K-Neighbour and Logistic Regression where we have calculated Precision, Recall, F-1 Score and Accuracy of each ML algorithms mentioned earlier. We observed that we are getting better accuracy in Random Forest Classifier as compared to the work that was proposed earlier.

Table 9.2 consists of Precision, Recall, F-1 score and Accuracy, which are calculated when we have applied Particle Swarm Optimization technique in Random Forest Classifier, Support Vector Machine and XgBoost Classifier. After successfully applying these, we have observed that as compared to Random Forest in Table 9.1 we are getting better accuracy, an obtained accuracy of 83.92%.

TABLE 9.1
Proposed Method Accuracy Using ML Algorithms Where We Are Getting Better Accuracy with Random Forest, XgBoost and NuSVC (Nu Support Vector Classifier)

S.No	Methods	Precision	Recall	F-1 Score	Accuracy %
1.	Random Forest	80	82	83	81.5
2.	Support Vector Machine	71	68	77	77.00
3.	Decision Tree Classifier	75	77	80	76.77
4.	XgBoost	80	82	82	83.2
5.	Adaboost Classifier	80.5	80	80	80.3
6.	K-Neighbour Classifier	69	67	67	66.96
7.	Logistic Regression	75	74	74	74.10
8.	NuSVC	81	80	80	80.35

TABLE 9.2
Proposed Methods with PSO Optimization Where We Are Getting Maximum Accuracy of 83.92% with Random Forest Algorithm

S.No	Method	Precision	Recall	F-1 Score	Accuracy (%)
1.	Random Forest	84	84	83.5	83.92
2.	SVM	80	78	78	77.67
3.	XgBoost	83	83	83	83.03

Table 9.3 compares variation of SVM. It consists of Normal SVC, Nu-SVC, and Linear SVC and for all variations of SVM we have calculated Precision, Recall, F1-Score and Accuracy. We are calculating these because we wanted to be sure which SVM is giving the best results. From the below table we can conclude that NuSVC is giving the better result, with a 80.35% accuracy.

TABLE 9.3
Performance of Various SVM Classifier, Getting Maximum Accuracy of 80.32% with NuSVC (Nu Support Vector Classifier)

S.No.	SVM Type	Precision	Recall	F1-Score	Accuracy (%)
1.	Normal SVC	80	78	78	77.67
2.	NuSVC	81	80	80	80.35
3.	Linear SVC	75	67	63	66.96

Table 9.4 consists of parameters of Random Forest Classifier, namely n-estimator, max-depth and max-feature. With the variation of these parameters we are trying to obtain the best accuracy for Random Forest. Therefore, in the below table we are putting n-estimator constant for calculating accuracy and we have observed that we are getting 83.92% of accuracy for n-estimator of 200.

Table 9.5 consists of parameters of Random Forest Classifier which is n-estimator, max-depth and max-feature and with the variation of these parameters we are trying to get the best accuracy for Random Forest. Therefore, in the table below we are putting max-depth constant for calculating accuracy and we have observed that we are getting 85.70% of accuracy for n-estimator of 75 and a max-feature of 8.

TABLE 9.4
Parameter Tuning in Random Forest Classifier Putting n-estimator and Max Feature Constant Where We Are Getting Maximum Accuracy of 83.92%

S.No.	n-estimator	max-depth	Max-feature	Accuracy (%)
1.	200	4	auto	78.57
2.	200	5	auto	78.57
3.	200	6	auto	81.25
4.	200	7	auto	83.03
5.	200	8	auto	83.92
6.	200	9	auto	83.03

The best accuracy found for n-estimator = 200, max-depth = 8, max-feature = auto is 83.92%.

TABLE 9.5
Parameter Tuning in Random Forest Classifier Putting Max-depth and Max-feature Constant Where We Are Getting Maximum Accuracy of 85.70%

S. No.	n-estimator	max-depth	Max-feature	Accuracy (%)
1.	10	8	auto	80.03
2.	30	8	auto	84.82
3.	50	8	auto	83.92
4.	70	8	auto	84.82
5.	75	8	auto	85.70
6.	76	8	auto	82.24
7.	90	8	auto	83.03

The best accuracy found for n-estimator = 75, max-depth = 8, max-feature = auto is 85.70%.

TABLE 9.6
Comparison of Random Forest and Support Vector Machine between Previous Work and Proposed Method Where We Are Getting Better Result in Random Forest Algorithm

S.No.	Name of Author	Method Name	Precision	Recall	F1-Score	Accuracy (%)
1.	Tong et al. [7]	Random Forest	—	86.7	—	80.7
2.	Proposed	Random Forest	84	84	83.5	85.70
3.	Beheshti et al. [4]	SVM	—	80.20	—	84.90
4.	Proposed	SVM	81	80	80	80.35

9.6 DISCUSSION

Table 9.6 shows a comparison of Random Forest and Support Vector machine in previous work and our proposed method where we are getting better results in the Random Forest Algorithm.

From the comparison we can see that the method that is proposed by Tong et al. [7] achieves an accuracy of 80.7, which is a lower accuracy than in the method that we have proposed. Our proposed method Random Forest Classifier achieves accuracy of 85.70%. This accuracy was achieved using Particle Swarm Optimization Technique followed by tuning the parameter of Random Forest Classifier.

9.7 CONCLUSION

In this paper, we have proposed a Particle Swarm Optimization machine learning algorithm for prediction of Alzheimer's disease. In our methods we have used dataset provided by ADNI for machine learning models and we have used seven machine learning models; namely Support Vector Machine Classification, Random Forest Classification, XgBoost Classifier, Decision Tree Classification, Adaboost Classifier, K-Neighbour Classifier and Logistic Regression and an accuracy of 80.35, 85.71%, 83.92%, 76.77%, 80.3%, 66.96% and 74.10% is achieved, respectively. Notice that our proposed method obtains an accuracy of 85.71% for classification of patients as Dementia and Non-Dementia. In future work, will investigate the combination of Deep Learning methods with Particle Swarm Optimization technique to further improve accuracy and dynamic analysis of the results.

REFERENCES

1. Almasi, Omid Naghash, Ehsan Akhtarshenas, and Modjtaba Rouhani. "An efficient model selection for SVM in real-world datasets using BGA and RGA." *Neural Network World* 24.5 (2014): 501.
2. Zhang, Daoqiang, Dinggang Shen, and Alzheimer's Disease Neuroimaging Initiative. "Multi-modal multi-task learning for joint prediction of multiple regression and classification variables in Alzheimer's disease." *NeuroImage* 59.2 (2012): 895–907.

3. Mareeswari, S., and G. Wiselin Jiji. "A survey: early detection of Alzheimer's disease using different techniques." *International Journal of Computer Science and Applications* 5.1 (2015): 27–37.
4. Spulber, Gabriela, et al. "An MRI-based index to measure the severity of Alzheimer's disease-like structural pattern in subjects with mild cognitive impairment." *Journal of Internal Medicine* 273.4 (2013): 396–409.
5. Westman, Eric, et al. "AddNeuroMed and ADNI: similar patterns of Alzheimer's atrophy and automated MRI classification accuracy in Europe and North America." *Neuroimage* 58.3 (2011): 818–828.
6. Beheshti, Iman, et al. "Classification of Alzheimer's disease and prediction of mild cognitive impairment-to-Alzheimer's conversion from structural magnetic resource imaging using feature ranking and a genetic algorithm." *Computers in Biology and Medicine* 83 (2017): 109–119.
7. Tong, Tong, et al. "A novel grading biomarker for the prediction of conversion from mild cognitive impairment to Alzheimer's disease." *IEEE Transactions on Biomedical Engineering* 64.1 (2016): 155–165.
8. Rajeesh, Jayapathy, Rama Swamy Moni, and Thankappan Gopalakrishnan. "Discrimination of Alzheimer's disease using hippocampus texture features from MRI." *Asian Biomedicine* 6.1 (2012): 87–94.
9. Zhang, Yu-Dong, Shuihua Wang, and Zhengchao Dong. "Classification of Alzheimer disease based on structural magnetic resonance imaging by kernel support vector machine decision tree." *Progress in Electromagnetics Research* 144 (2014): 171–184.
10. Yang, Shih-Ting, et al. "Discrimination between Alzheimer's disease and mild cognitive impairment using SOM and PSO-SVM." *Computational and Mathematical Methods in Medicine* 2013 (2013): 1–10.
11. Sweety, M. Evanchalin, and G. Wiselin Jiji. "Detection of Alzheimer disease in brain images using PSO and Decision Tree Approach." *2014 IEEE International Conference on Advanced Communications, Control and Computing Technologies*. IEEE, 2014.
12. Zhang, Yudong, et al. "An MR brain images classifier system via particle swarm optimization and kernel support vector machine." *The Scientific World Journal* 2013 (2013): 1–9.
13. Sivapriya, T. R., A. R. Nadira Banu Kamal, and V. Thavavel. "Automated classification of dementia using PSO based least square support vector machine." *International Journal of Machine Learning and Computing* 3.2 (2013): 181.
14. S. KumarPandey and R. RamJanghel, "A survey on missing information strategies and imputation methods in healthcare," 2018 8th International Conference on Cloud Computing, Data Science & Engineering (Confluence), Noida, 2018, pp. 299–304.
15. https://towardsdatascience.com/feature-engineering-for-machine-learning-3a5e293a5114#ad97.
16. https://www.geeksforgeeks.org/ml-label-encoding-of-datasets-in-python/
17. Binitha, S., and S. Siva Sathya. "A survey of bio inspired optimization algorithms." *International Journal of Soft Computing and Engineering* 2.2 (2012): 137–151.
18. https://www.datacamp.com/community/tutorials/random-forests-classifier-python.
19. https://towardsdatascience.com/support-vector-machine-introduction-to-machine-learning-algorithms-934a444fca47.
20. https://dataaspirant.com/2017/01/30/how-decision-tree-algorithm-works/.
21. https://www.analyticsvidhya.com/blog/2018/09/an-end-to-end-guide-to-understand-the-math-behind-xgboost/.
22. https://medium.com/machine-learning-101/https-medium-com-savanpatel-chapter-6-adaboost-classifier-b945f330af06.

10 Parkinson's Disease Detection Using Voice Measurements

Raj Kumar Patra, Akanksha Gupta, Maguluri Sudeep Joel, and Swati Jain

CONTENTS

10.1 INTRODUCTION

Venture's fundamental point is to distinguish Parkinson's syndrome utilizing basic AI algorithms to anticipate progressively exact and applicable forecasts with less time and cost as there is a great deal of open source information available of perceptions of individuals having Parkinson's syndrome [1].

10.2 LITERATURE SURVEY

A literature survey has been created to abrogate the issues winning in the rehearsing manual framework. The activities carried out in the manual framework take additional time as they rely upon progressive clinical testing requiring administrative work. We have to build up a computerized framework where we can without too much difficulty distinguish the syndrome and take preventive measures before it reaches an advanced stage. There is no specific method of testing (for example, blood or urine) the presence of the syndrome. The best way to distinguish it is by studying the indications and conducting an examination. It is a major undertaking to look at and break down the human voice. Therefore, the vocal chronicles are partitioned into a couple of significant highlights to recognize the degree of jitter and sparkling in the voice. These highlights are scaled up to prepare the model to utilize an outfit classifier. For example, XGBoost classifier is an increasingly proficient and powerful approach to prepare a model and it utilizes decision trees [2].

10.2.1 Parkinson's Syndromes

Parkinson syndrome could be dynamic framework nervous disorder which influence movements of individuals. Symptoms may start continuously, or here and there or as a hardly perceptible tremor in a hand. Tremors are typical; however, confusion likewise typically caused firmness or facilitation back of growth. In the initial phases of Parkinson's syndrome the face might not show any signs. Arms probably won't swing while walking [3]. The voice may or nay not turn out to be faint or slurred. Parkinson's syndrome side effects compound as the condition progresses. Despite the fact that Parkinson's syndrome can't be fixed, medication might help with its indications. Periodically, primary care physicians will recommend medical means to deal with issues connected to specific districts of the cerebrum and improve side effects.

10.2.2 Symptoms

Parkinson's syndrome indications and consequences might vary widely. Primary signs are often mild and go undetected. Symptoms regularly appear on a single side of the body and remain more pronounced on that side; often side effects later begin to impact both sides of body.

Tremors/shaking. Tremors as a rule begins in an appendage, typically on hands or fingers. Individual may rub their thumb and index-finger back and forth, kown as a pill-moving tremor. The hand might tremor while the individual is motionless [4–6].

Slowness of movement (bradykinesia). Later, Parkinson's syndrome might slow down movement, making straightforward tasks difficult and tedious. One's steps will become smaller when walking and it may become difficult to get up from a seated position. individual might falter while attempting walking. Unbending muscle fibres. Muscular inflexibility or cramps occurred in one body parts randomly. Hardened muscles cause difficulties and limit the span of movements [7].

Impeded position, balance and automatic movment. Position might be deformed, or there may be balance challenges caused by Parkinson's syndrome. Decrease in automatic movement. One might have lessened capacity to control movment such as arms swinging, squinting, grinning and so forth. Voice changes. One might talk precisely or rapidy, slur or hesitate while/before speaking or talking. Voice might become monotone without the usual enunciations.

10.2.3 Causes

Parkinson's syndrome causes neurons, the nervous cells of brain, to break down and die. Major consequences result from the death of neurons that produce a chemical carrier in our brain know as Dopamine. Once dopamine levels are reduced in the brain, irregular brain functioning provokes the side effects of Parkinson's syndrome. The real cause of Parkinson's syndrome is obscure; however, a few factors appear to be key in this condition, including:

- **Genes:** Researchers have distinguished obvious hereditary factors in Parkinson's syndrome. However, these are rare and it is unusual for numerous persons of the same family to have Parkinson's syndrome symptoms. Yet a few gene traits seem to increase the chances of Parkinson's syndrome, with moderately less chances of Parkinson's syndrome for every one of these marked genes.
- **Ecological activates:** Contact with certain poisons or biological variables might increase the the risk of future Parkinson's syndrome, yet the threat is moderately lower.
  Researchers likewise observed a number of variations in the brain of person influenced by Parkinson's syndrome, notwithstanding the fact that it's unclear what causes these alterations. These include [8]:
- **Existence of Lewy bodies:** Clusters of particular compounds in synapses are relatively small indicators of Parkinson's syndrome. These are known as Lewy bodies, and investigators accept that these figures indicate a cause of Parkinson's syndrome [9].
- **Alpha-synuclein found within Lewy bodies:** As several compounds are located in Lewy bodies, scientists find noteworthy a protein called alpha-synuclein (a-synuclein). It is initiated within Lewy bodies in a combined structure that doesn't let the cells detach. This is now a very important subject of focus amongst Parkinson's syndrome scientists [10].

10.2.4 Threat Causes

Risk factors for Parkinson's syndrome include:

- **Age:** Young adults every so often experience Parkinson's syndrome, but it conventionally commences after midlife and the risk rises as one gets older. Persons normally start experiencing the syndrome at age 60 or later [11].
- **Heredity:** With close relatives having Parkinson's syndrome the probability that an individual may also be affected by the syndrome increases. However, the possibility is still very small except in instances where there are a number of family members with Parkinson's syndrome.
- **Sex:** Males are more likely to be affected by Parkinson's syndrome than Females.

10.2.5 Complications

Some complications frequently associated with Parkinson's syndrome [11–16]:

- **Thinking:** Those with Parkinson's syndrome might encounter intellectual difficulties (dementia) and thinking challenges. This normally happens in a later phase of Parkinson's syndrome. Such psychological concerns are not very receptive to prescriptions.
- **Depression and emotional changes:** Person with Parkinson's syndrome may encounter depression, in some cases in the initial phases. This may be managed with treament. Persons with Parkinson's syndrome may likewise face further emotional changes; for example, loss of motivation, fear or nervousness. Doctors can prescribe prescriptions to treat these manifestations.
- **Swallowing problems:** People with Parkinson's syndrome can experience problems in swallowing as their illness increases. Saliva accumulating in the patient's mouth because of eased back swallowing may prompt salivating.
- **Chewing and eating problems:** In later stages Parkinson's syndrome impacts muscles in the patient's mouth, resulting in chewing problems, gagging and lack of nutrition.
- **Sleep problem and sleep disorders:** Individuals affected by Parkinson's syndrome regularly experience sleep issues, ranging from becoming awakened every now and then, being awake the entire whole night, awakening earlier or falling asleep in the day time. Individuals may similarly face quick eye movement sleeping problems, including hallucinations. Medication can assist patients with sleeping disorders.
- **Bladder problems:** Parkinson's syndrome may also trigger bladder issues, involving not being able to control urine or experiencing trouble while urinating.
- **Constipation Problem:** Many individuals affected by Parkinson's syndrome experience constipation, fundamentally as of a slow stomach digestion.

10.3 METHODOLOGIES USED IN PRESENT WORK

Objectives:

- Artificial Intelligence (AI) and comprehend its relationship with information.

- Machine Learning (ML) and comprehend its relationship with Artificial Intelligence.
- Machine Learning approach and its relationship with data science.
- Identify the application.

Definition of Artificial Intelligence:

Artificial Intelligence alludes to insight showed by machines that simulates human intelligence.

The Emergence of Artificial Intelligence:

The data economy and its large stores are allowing remarkable advancement in the data science field, mining valuable data and comprehension from existing information. Data science is moving towards a new worldview where individuals can instruct machines/computers to acquire knowledge from available data and determine a range of valuable knowledge. That is called Artificial Intelligence (AI).

AI in Practice:

Listed below are some examples where AI is utilized broadly in this Machine Learning instructional exercise.

- Self driving automobiles
- Artificial Assistants like Google Assistant, Siri that listen and answers to the human voice
- AlphaGo Artificial assistant of Google that has beaten many Go champs, for example, Ke Jie
- Applying Artificial Intelligence in chess
- Amazon home control chatbot gadget i.e., ECHO
- Hilton consuming Connie – concierge robot from IBM Watson

Data Facilitates Artificial Intelligence Products:

Amazon fetches data and information from its customer's database to suggest items to customers. This feature attracts more customers. Then, more consumers generate more data which helps improve the suggestions significantly.

Machine Learning:

Proficiency in the "Artificial Intelligence" framework to grasp knowledge by extricating designs from data is called Machine Learning.

Benefits of Machine Learning:

- Powerful Processing
- Better Prediction Ability and Decision Making
- Rapid Processing
- Accuracy
- Affordable Management of Data
- Economical
- Complex Big Data Analysis

Features of Machine Learning:

- Machine Learning is computing concentrated and requires significantly large amounts of training and data/information
- It comprises routine training to increase knowledge, learning and decision-making capabilities of the system.
- As new data is integrated, Machine Learning training can be automatedd for learning new data designs/patterns and enhancing its computation.

Model: Learning from new spam words or a new Voice (likewise called gradual learning)

10.3.1 Machine Learning (ML) and Artificial Intelligence (AI)

ML (machine learning) is a methodology or subclass of AI (Artificial Intelligence) that depends on the possibility that machinery can offer access to information alongside the capacity to gain knowledge from it.

Traditional Programming versus a Machine Learning Approach Traditional programming depends on hard-coded rules.

Machine Learning depends on learning designs dependent on test information.

As you go from rule-based frameworks to those of profound learning, progressively complex highlights and iinformation yield connections become learnable.

- Data Science and Machine Learning are connected at the hip. Information Science assesses information for Machine Learning calculations.
- Data science is the utilization of factual strategies to discover designs in the information.
- Statistical ML utilizes indistinguishable math and strategies from information science.
- These methods are coordinated into calculations that learn and enhance their own.
- Machine Learning encourages Artificial Intelligence as it empowers machines to gain from the examples in information.

Machine Learning Techniques:

1. Classification
2. Categorization
3. Grouping
4. Trend examination
5. Anomaly recognition
6. Visualization
7. Decision creation

Machine Learning Algorithms:

Let us comprehend Machine Learning Algorithms in detail.

- Machine Learning can gain from named information (known as regulated learning) or unlabelled information (known as unaided learning).
- Machine Learning calculations including unlabelled information, or solo learning, are more convoluted than those with the named information or managed learning.
- Machine Learning calculations can be utilized to settle on choices in the emotional realm also.

Models:

- Logistic Regression can be utilized to anticipate which gathering will succeed at the polling station.
- Naïve Bayes calculation can isolate legitimate messages from spam.

Applications of Machine Learning:

Some uses and application of ML (Machine learning) are referenced below.

- Image Processing
- Robotics
- Data Mining
- Video Games
- Text Analysis
- Healthcare

Applications:

Image Processing:

- Image labelling and acknowledgment
- Self-driving vehicles
- Optical Character Recognition (OCR)

Robotics:

- Human re-enactment
- Industrial apply autonomy

Data Mining:

- Anomaly identification
- Grouping and predictions
- Association rules

Text Analysis:

- Sentiment analysis
- Spam filtering
- Information extraction

10.3.2 Ensemble Learning

Slope Boosting Machines fit into a classification of ML called Ensemble Learning, which is a part of ML strategies that prepare and foresee numerous models quickly to deliver a single predominant yield.

Group learning is separated into three essential subsets:

- Bagging
- Stacking
- Boosting

Ensemble learning as shown in Figure 10.1 is the procedure by which numerous prototypes like, classifiers and specialists are deliberately made and consolidated to tackle a specific computational knowledge issue. Gathering learning is principally used to enhance (grouping, forecast, probability, estimation etc.) the implementation of a model, or reduce the possibility of a shocking determination of a worthless one. Different uses of ensemble learning integrate allocating a certainty to the conclusion made by the model, deciding optimal (or close to optimal) highlights, data fusion, steady learning, nonstationary learning and mistake adjusting. This article centers around grouping related to uses of outfit learning; nonethelss, all standard thoughts depicted below can be handily summed up to work with estimate or forecast type issues also.

1. **Bagging:** Bagging attempts to actualize comparable students on little example populaces and afterward takes a mean of the considerable number of expectations. In sum, with packing you one can utilize various students on various populaces. As one may anticipate, this should decrease fluctuation error.

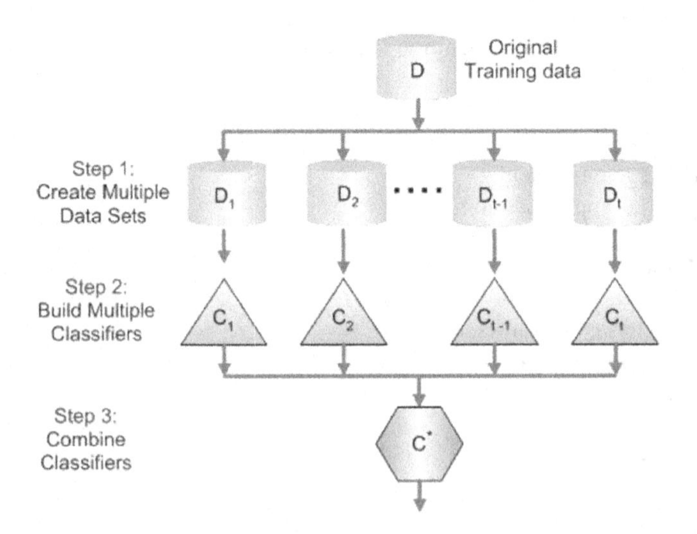

FIGURE 10.1 Graphical Representation of Multiple Classifiers.

2. **Boosting:** Boosting is an iterative method which change the heaviness of a perception dependent on the last characterization as depicted in the Figure 10.2. In the event that a perception was characterized mistakenly, it attempts to expand the heaviness of this perception and vice-versa. Boosting all in all abatements the predisposition blunder and constructs solid prescient models. However, they may occasionally overfit on the preparation information.
3. **Stacking:** This is an exceptionally fascinating method of joining models as shown in Figure 10.3. Here we utilize a student to consolidate yield from various students. This can prompt diminishing in either predisposition or fluctuation blunder contingent upon the consolidating student we use.

XGBoost Classifier: XGBoost is a famous procedure and a slick option in contrast to customary relapse or neural webs. It represents EXtreme Gradient Enhancing, and basically approximately constructs a decision tree to register angles as depicted in Figure 10.4. Figure 10.4 illustrates a well-known detail from the XGBoost site.

This sounds straightforward, yet can be very potent. Take, for example, Parkinson recognition: we have numerous measurements that we can break down and eventually we have to identify Parkinson's (arrangement!). This is an ideal issue for XGBoost (particularly as there is a solitary yield so we do not have to

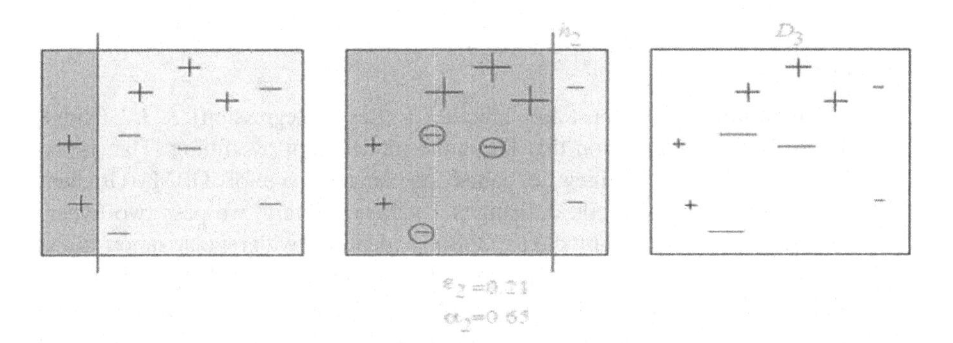

FIGURE 10.2 Boosting.

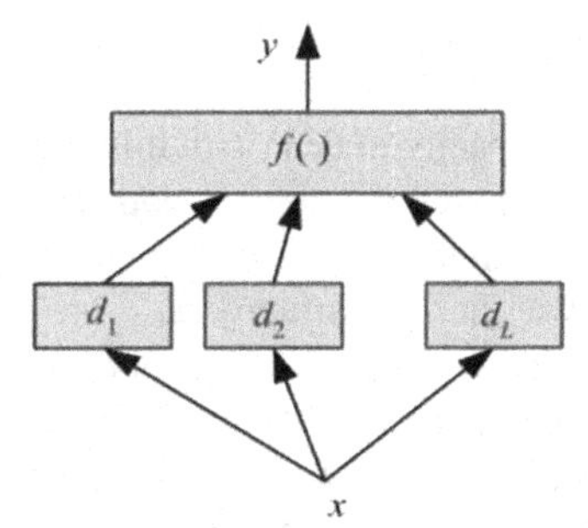

FIGURE 10.3 Stacking.

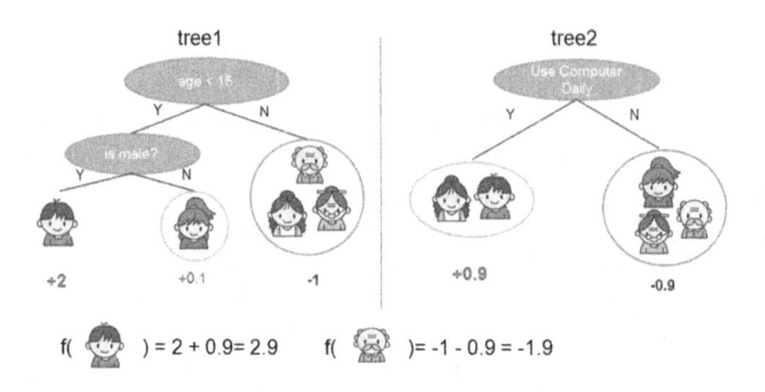

FIGURE 10.4 Example of Parkinson Detection.

apply Multioutput wrapper, about which more will be said later). XGBoosting is amazing and can be a valuable device for Patient's next venture! XGBoosting goes a lot further, howeve—for various yields you do require Multioutput model (SciKit Learn takes an incredible covering for this), and for increasingly precise fetching you will have to calibrate Patient's XGBoost model. In Jupiter notepad previously (and in a repository attached underneath) we investigate utilizing Keras aimed at the ceaseless facts, yet Multioutput wrapping from sklearn can almost serve as a drop-in substitute for the Keras model.

10.3.3 Advantages

1. **Regularization:** XGBoost has inbuilt L1 (Lasso Regression) & L2 (Ridge Regression) regularization that keeps the model from overfitting. That is the reason, XGBoost is likewise called regularized type of GBM (Gradient Boosting Machine). While utilizing Scikit Learn library, we pass two hyper-boundaries (alpha and lambda) to XGBoost identified with regularization. alpha is utilized for L1 regularization and lambda is utilized for L2 regularization.
2. **Parallel Processing:** XGBoost uses intensity of parallel processing and that's the reason it is lot speedier than GBM. It utilizes different CPU centers to execute the model. While utilizing Scikit Learn library, nthread hyper-boundary is utilized for equal handling. nthread speaks to number of CPU centers to be utilized. If one wanted to employ all the accessible cores, but did not specify an incentive for nthread, the calculation would identify consequently.
3. **Missing Value Handling:** XGBoost has inbuilt capacity to deal with missing qualities. While XGBoost experiences a missing node, it attempts both left and right-hand split and learns the path, prompting higher loss for every node. It at that point does likewise when chipping away at the testing data.
4. **Cross Validation:** XGBoost permits clients to track cross-approval by each cycle of boosting procedure; and in this manner it is simple to develop the specific ideal amount of boosting repetitions in a solitary outing. This is unlike all GBM, where one need to execute grid search and just constrained worth can be tried.
5. **Effective Tree Pruning:** A GBM may quit parting nodes once it experiences

an undesirable damage in splitting. Subsequently, it is even further a desirous algorithm. XGBoost then again makes fragments up to max_depth determined and afterward starts trimming a tree backwards and eliminates splitting outside, which there is no optimistic achievement.

10.3.4 Data Drive Machine Learning

As significant amounts of data is accessible, we have enhanced data to present to the patients. Predictive algo and AI can provide us an excellent predictive model of death which can be used by doctors and specialists to instruct patients.

However, ML (Machine Learning) needs definite quantity of data to produce powerful algorithms. A lot of ML (Machine Learning) will primarily originate from associations with enormous data-sets. Wellbeing Catalyst is creating Collective Analytics for Excellence (CAFÉ™), an application based on a national de-recognized storehouse of social insurance information from big business information distribution centres (EDWs) and third-party information sources. It is empowering relative viability, research, and creating interesting, incredible AI calculations. Bistro gives a joint effort among our medicinal services framework accomplices, of all shapes and sizes. Research, and creating one-of -a-kind, ground-breaking AI calculations. Bistro provides a joint effort among our social insurance framework accomplices, of all shapes and sizes.

10.3.5 Architecture

The underneath architecture in Figure 10.5 shows the strategy followed for ailment recognition utilizing AI, beginning from contribution to definite forecast.

Input Data: Input information is by and large in.csv configuration or information group where the information is brought and planned in the information confined from the source sections.

Reading Data: Pandas library is utilized to add the information to the information outline.

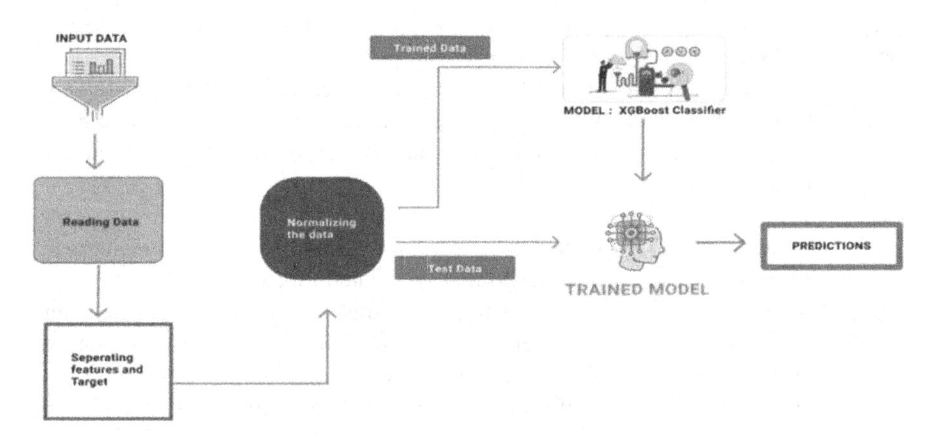

FIGURE 10.5 Flow Diagram of Proposed Worked.

Separating Features and Targets: We are going to isolate the highlights which we take to preparing the model by giving the objective worth for example 1/0 for the specific blend of highlights.

Normalization: Normalization is a significant advance while we are dealing with huge qualities in the highlights, as the higher piece whole numbers will cost high computational force and time. To accomplish the effectiveness in calculation we will standardize the information esteems.

Test Data and Training: Training information is passed to XGBoost classifier to prepare models. Test information is then utilized to test the prepared models, whether it is making right forecasts or not.

XGBoost Classifier: The reason for picking the XGXGBboost classifier for this undertaking is the effectiveness and exactness that we have seen when contrasted with different classifiers. At last, we breeze through the assessment information to the prepared model case to make expectations.

System Analysis is the significant stage in process of system development. System investigators perform the significant job of interrogator and dwell profoundly on the working of the current system. In study, a point by point examination of these activities implemented by system and their contacts inside and outside the system is over. The main inquiry arising here is, "what must be done to take care of the problem"? As the most widely recognized neurodegenerative development issue, Parkinson's Syndrome (PD) has an enormous effect on medicinal service frameworks around the globe. While customarily much accentuation has been put on the engine parts of the illness, it is progressively perceived that PD is a multisystem issue, and huge numbers of the non-engine highlights play as significant a role in affecting general personal satisfaction. There are various new advances that may enormously aid early determination, checking and treatment of this condition. Current neuroimaging advancements, including MRI, EEG, MEG, PET, and CT scan noninvasively look at the ailing mind and research the fundamental neural frameworks in PD, bringing about amazing methodologies for illness recognition and observing. New information combination strategies can join data from reciprocal innovations taking into account far reaching evaluations. New light-weight and remote sensors can screen development, electrodermal reactions, temperature and pulse. Non-intrusive electrical incitement can balance cerebrum action, providing new unexplored avenues of treatment.

So as to have a diagram of new advances in PD research and make a step towards examining how these can be utilized to survey and treat PD. For this research topic, we are interested in unique explorations. Potential subtopics incorporate yet are not restricted to the following:

- Biomarkers of PD dependent on auxiliary or utilitarian minitrial incitement.
- Data fusion strategies relevant to malady related biodata.
- Motion Biomarkers Shows Extreme Contrast amongst Fit Subjects and Parkinson's Syndrome Patients Cured by Deep Brain Stimulation of Subthalamic Nucleus. A Preliminary Study
- Adjustments of Local Uniformity in Parkinson's Syndrome Patients by Icing of Gait: A Resting-State fMRI Study

- Altered Global Synchronizations in Patients by Parkinson's Syndrome: A Resting-State fMRI Study

10.4 PROPOSED SYSTEM

Utilizing AI calculations, we can accomplish Parkinson's ailment discovery with much fitting outcomes in less time and cost utilizing amazing, vigorous and productive classifiers accessible utilizing choice trees.

Details of the Data-set:

Source:

The data-set was built through "Max little" of "University of Oxford," as a team by the National Centre for Opinion & Communication, Denver, CO, who recorded the Voice indications.

The first analysis distributed the feature removal techniques for common speech issue.

Data-Set Evidence:

This dataset is made out of a scope of bio-medical speech assessment starting with 31 individuals, 23 affected by Parkinson's syndrome (PS). Every segment in the table retains specific speech measure, and every line compares 1 of 195 speech recordings from these individuals ("name" section). The fundamental point of data is to separate sound individuals from those with PD, as indicated by the "status" section which is fixed to 0 for healthy and 1 for PD.

Attributes of the Data Used:

Name -ASCII subject name	MDVP: Flicker
MDVP: Fo (Hz)-Avg vocal	MDVP: Flicker(dB)
MDVP: Fhi (Hz)-Max vocal	Flicker: APQ3
MDVP: Flo (Hz)-Min vocal	Flicker: APQ5
MDVP: Jitter(%)	Flicker: DDA-Several measures of deviation in amplitude
MDVP: Jitter (Abs)	NHR, HNR-Two events of ratio of noise to tonal components in the speech
MDVP:RAP	RPDE, D2-Two nonlinear dynamical difficulty events
MDVP: PPQ	DFA-Signal fractal scaling exponent spread1,spread2,PPE
MDVP: APQ	status-Health status of the subject (one)-Parkinson(zero)-healthy
Jitter: DDP-Several measures of variation in fundamental frequency	

Relation between prominent features and status variable:

- Figure 10.6 shows that RPDE (i.e. a non-linear dynamical complexity measure) VS The status of the patient (0–healthy and 1–Syndrome).
- HNR is a measure of ratio of noise to tonal components in the voice VS.
- The status of the patient (0–healthy and 1–Syndrome).

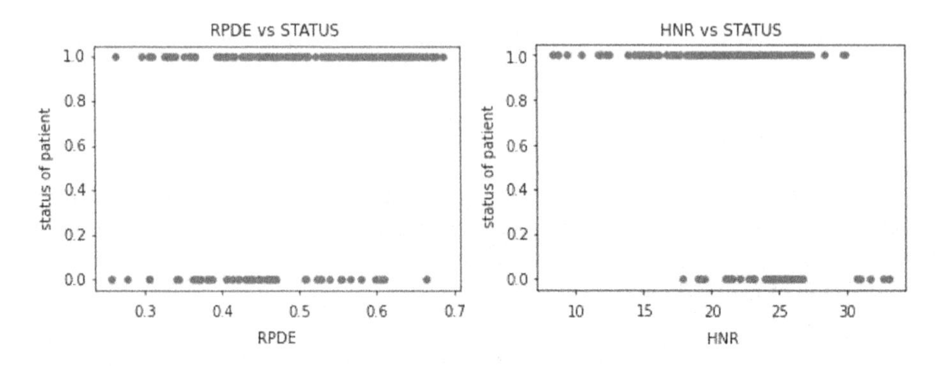

FIGURE 10.6 Relation Between Prominent Features and Status Variable.

The probability of undertaking is examined in this segment and a strategic plan remains advanced with a broad arrangement for task and about cost quotes. During system examination the possibility study of the proposed framework remains to be completed. This remains to guarantee that the anticipated structure isn't a liability to the organization. Three key observations associated with the Probability Study are:

1. Economic Probability
2. Social Probability
3. Technical Probability

Economic Probability:

The study is done to check the fiscal effect that the outline will have on the lodgings. The amount of assets that inns can fill pioneering work of the system is circumscribed. These usages need to be supported.

Technical Probability:

The study is done to check technological probability, which remains the technological fundamentals of structure. Any of the arrangement generated must not have an appeal on existing technological assets. The built system must have a retiring requirement, as minor or void variations are vital for applying this organization.

Social Probability:

This study is to determine the degree of acceptance of this structure by the consumer. It contains the way to reacting customer to his solicitation effectively. The consumer must not sense faltered, rather should acknowledge it as a need.

10.5 TESTING

The motive for testing is to detect faults. It remains a mode to discover each possible error or deficiency. It offers a method to form the effectiveness of segments, subassemblies, and assemblages ,as well as a finalized article. It remains a method of performing encoding with the objective of promising that the Software system lives up to its consumers requirements and doesn't fall flat in an inadmissible means. There are many kinds of tests. Every type tends to a particular testing criterion.

10.5.1 Type of Testing

Unit testing comprises the idea of experimentation that the internal program foundation is appropriately functioning and program inputs produce extensive output. Entire conclusion branches and interior codes must be authenticated. It is a testing of individual programming units of the software. Unit testing is done once a specific unit is completed before combination. This is a generic testing, which depends on information on its building and is insensitive. Unit tests implement necessary tests at part level and tests specific corporate procedures and software, as well as system arrangements. Unit tests promise that all remarkable means of a business procedure performs correctly to recorded particulars and comprises visibly categorized inputs and anticipated conclusions.

10.5.2 Integration Testing

Integration tests are planned to check combined programming fragments to check whether they run as a single application. Testing is case obsessed and is increasingly apprehensive about fundamental outcomes of shades or fields. Reconciliation tests show that despite the fact that the parts were independently fulfilled, as shown by efficient unit testing, the mix of parts is accurate and steady. Integration testing is explicitly planned for detecting the errors that appear from fusion of parts.

10.5.3 Functional Testing

Functional tests arranged show that capabilities tried are reachable as specified by business and technical needs, system documentation, and user's manuals.

Functional testing includes the accompanying points:

- Valid input: diagnosed lessons of valid enter have to be well-known.
- Invalid input: diagnosed instructions of invalid enter should be rejected.
- Capabilities: identified features have to be exercised.
- Output: recognized instructions of utility outputs must be exercised.
- Systems/approaches: interfacing structures or techniques have to be invoked.

10.6 CONCLUSION AND FUTURE ENHANCEMENTS

In this Python AI venture, we figured out how to identify the advance of Parkinson's syndrome in people utilizing different variables. We utilized an XGB Classifier and utilized sklearn library to set up the data-set. Which gives us an exactness of 94.871%, which is incredible, giveng the quantity of lines of code in this python development. Utilizing AI calculations, we can accomplish Parkinson's malady discovery with proper outcomes with exceptionally less time and cost, utilizing incredible, strong and productive classifiers accessible utilizing choice trees. We will stack data, get highlights and names, scale highlights, at that point split data-set, construct a XGBClassifier, and afterward calculate the precision of our model.

Currently there is not any more productive data accessible as open source as the clinical industry's momentum research work is being done to fix the malady. To obtain increasingly precise expectations, a mass of information is required with additional highlights; i.e., as of now we are distinguishing this utilizing jitter and gleam in the voice. Later on we can likewise consider the standing situation of the patient utilizing picture preparing and considering a lot more side effects location turns out to be progressively productive. We can make this an open source by providing a web interface where the patient's information can be given as information and results will be obtained through the interface.

REFERENCES

1. Ada and Kaur, R., (2013), Early Detection and Prediction of Lung Cancer Survival Using Neural Network Classifier, *International Journal Of application or Innovation in Engineering and Management*, Vol. 2, No. 6, pp. 375–383.
2. Ada and Kaur, R., (2013), Feature Extraction and Principal Component Analysis for Lung Cancer Detection in CT Scan Images, *International Journal of Advanced Research in Computer Science and Software Engineering*, Vol. 3, pp. 187–190.
3. Ada, Kaur, R., (2013), Using Some Data Mining Technique to Predict the Survival Year of Lung Cancer Patient, *International Journal Of Computer Science and Mobile Computing*, Vol. 2, No. 4, pp. 1–6.
4. Aggarwal, P. and Kumar, R., (2013), Detection of Ground Glass Nodules in Human Lungs Using Lungs CT Scans Images, *International Journal of Current Engineering and Technology*, Vol. 3, No. 2, pp. 484–487.
5. Aggarwal, P., Vig, R. and Sardana, H. K., (2013), Semantic and Content-Based Medical Image Retrieval for Lung Cancer Diagnosis with the Inclusion of Expert Knowledge and Proven Pathology, Proceeding of IEEE Second International Conference on Image Information Processing, pp. 346–351.
6. Ajil, M. V. and Shreeram, S., (2015), Lung Cancer Detection from CT Image using Image Processing Techniques, *International Journal of Advance Research in Computer Science and Management Studies*, Vol. 3, No. 5, pp. 249–254.
7. Al-Ameen, Z., Al-Ameen, S., and Sulong, G., (2015), Latest Methods of Image Enhancement and Restoration for Computed Tomography: A Concise Review, *Applied Medical Informatics*, Vol. 36, No. 1, pp. 1–12.
8. Alavijeh, F. S., Nasab, H. M., (2014), Multi-scale Morphological Image Enhancement of Chest Radiographs by a Hybrid Scheme, *Journal of Medical Signals & Sensors*, Vol. 5, No. 1, pp. 59–68.
9. Al-Daoud, E., (2010), Cancer Diagnosis Using Modified Fuzzy Network, *Universal Journal of Computer Science and Engineering and Technology*, Vol. 1, pp. 73–78.
10. Al-Daoud, E., (2010), Cancer Diagnosis Using Modified Fuzzy Network, *Universal Journal of Computer Science and Engineering Technology*, Vol. 1, No. 2, pp. 73–78.
11. Al-Kadi, O. S., (2010), Assessment of Texture Measures Susceptibility to Noise in Conventional and Contrast Enhanced Computed Tomography Lung Tumours Images, *Computerized Medical Imaging and Graphics*, No. 34, pp. 494–503.
12. DATA: https://archive.ics.uci.edu/ml/machine-learning-databases/parkinsons/.
13. INSPIRATION: https://data-flair.training/.
14. DISEASE www.mayoclinic.org/diseases-conditions/parkinsons-disease/symptomscauses/.
15. XGBOOST https://towardsdatascience.com/exploring-xgboost-4baf9ace0cf6.
16. ENSEMBLE https://web.engr.oregonstate.edu/~tgd/publications/mcs-ensembles.pdf.

11 Speech Impairment Using Hybrid Model of Machine Learning

Renuka Arora, Sunny Arora, and Rishu Bhatia

CONTENTS

11.1 INTRODUCTION

Classification is a specific term in knowledge engineering and data mining. In learning techniques, classification gives an algorithmic process for creating a given input data into each other based on the different categories [1, 2]. Many real-time problems have been described as Classification Problems, for example, pattern recognition, medical diagnosis text categorization and many more. A classifier is an algorithm that utilizes classification-based results. The input data can be categorized with related classes. The characteristics of the classes can be described by a variety of features. These features can be of any type as integer-valued or real-valued. Classification is an example of a supervised learning procedure that is used to classify new knowledge-based factors. The result of learning patterns on various human affliction diagnoses supports medical specialists established on the effects of starting, even though some results exhibit the same factors [3–5]. One of the important multivariate technique problems is to choose specific characteristics from the basic attributes [6–8]. Clustering, Classification, Data processing, visualization and feature selection are various techniques supported by Python.

11.2 TYPES OF CLASSIFIER

Classification is a method to arrange the information into a required and special category value where labels can also be given to each category. There are several classifications uses as speech detection, biometric confirmation and document organization.

11.2.1 Naive Bayes (Classifier)

Naive Bayes may be a special classifier given by the Bayes theorem. There is an easy assumption in which conditionally autonomous attributes are used. The classification is categorized by deriving the theorem which is P(Ci|**X**) with a higher value than statement giving to Bayes theorem, as shown in Figure 11.1. This will reduce the price by including the categorized data. This data is valid as attributes are dependent and surprising.

11.2.2 Support Vector Machine (SVM)

The support vector machine is a version of the exercise data as points in space divided into classes by a crystal-clear gap that is as wide as required , as represented in Figure 11.2. New entries can also be used in that same space and related to a class based on which direction of the gap they drop. H1 is not a good hyperplane because of a separate class. H2 does but only with small value. H3 differentiates with effective distance factors of SVM.

11.2.3 K-Nearest Neighbor (KNN)

KNN gives an object by a bulk vote of the object's knowledge in the gap of the input values. The entity is given to the class which is most effective in their neighbor [4]. It is non-parametric because of no data distribution. It is lethargic since it does not study any pattern and build a simplification of the statistics as it

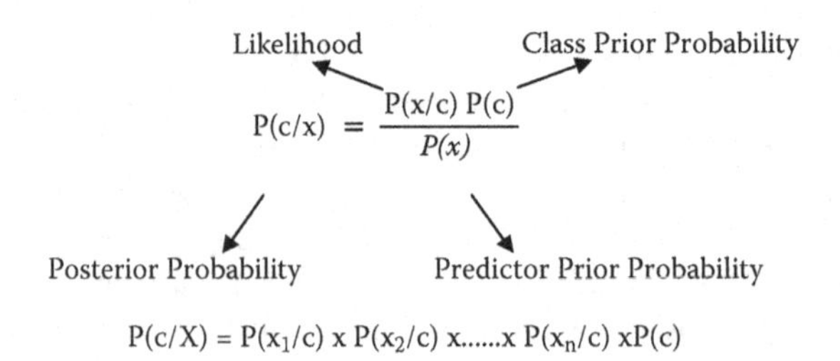

FIGURE 11.1 Naive Bayes Theorem.

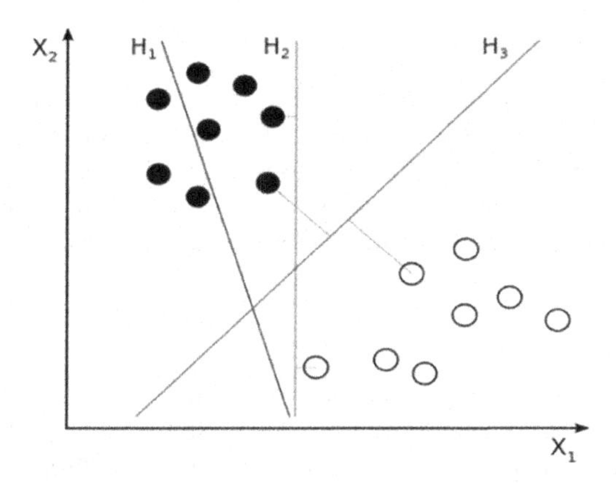

FIGURE 11.2 Support Vector Machine [5].

does not guide some values of some function where input X provides output y. So, it depends on the attribute similarity as an attribute is equal to input parameters. Classification is counted with the popular vote of the k nearest neighbors of each value, as shown in Figure 11.3.

11.2.4 Decision Tree

A decision tree gives a series of policies that can be used to organize the given statistics Decision Tree decides with a tree-structure model. It divides the section into two or more uniform sets based on the variations in your input data [3]. In this technique, the algorithm uses all characteristics and does a binary hole on definite data, crack by category and for continuous data a cut-off value is used. Select one value with low cost and effective incremental accuracy and repeats again and again, until maximum data depth is obtained as shown in Figure 11.4.

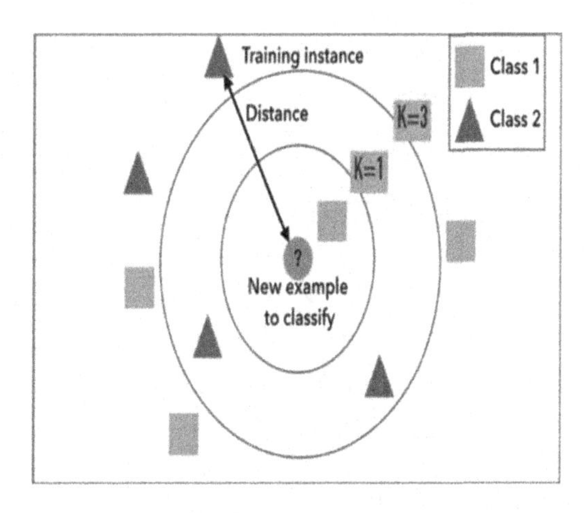

FIGURE 11.3 Classify New Example Depending on Training Instance Distance [5].

11.2.5 Random Forest

It is a pattern that increases with multiple trees and categorizes objects depending on the "votes" of all the trees, as shown in Figure 11.5. An object with high votes value is given to a class. This classifier uses many decision trees on datasets and uses average data to improve efficiency. The section size is always matched with the original input section size but the samples are shaped with substitution.

11.2.6 XGBoost

XGBoost is a decision-tree-like Machine algorithm that uses a boosting structure for definite and nonstop data. XGBoost is a precise functioning of incline boosting equipment and it has push limits of power for the algorithms. it was made and created for the pattern concert and increased speed, as shown in Figure 11.6.

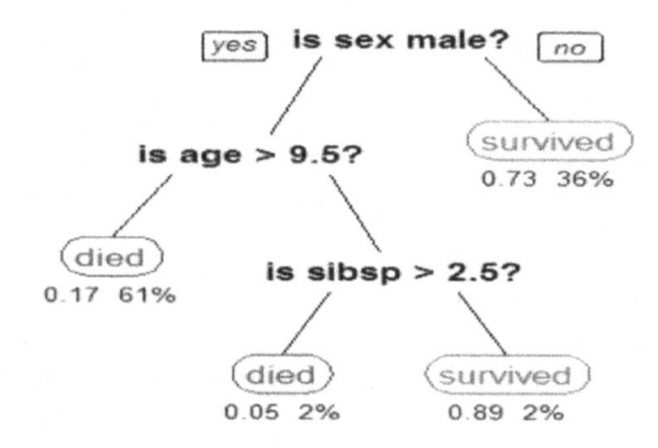

FIGURE 11.4 Tree-like Representations of Data in the Decision Tree [18].

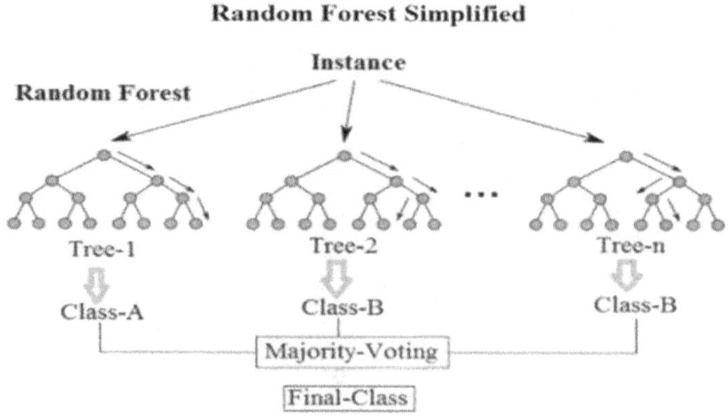

Random Forest Simplified
Instance
Random Forest
Tree-1
Tree-2
Tree-n
Class-A
Class-B
Class-B
Majority-Voting
Final-Class

FIGURE 11.5 Random Forest [21].

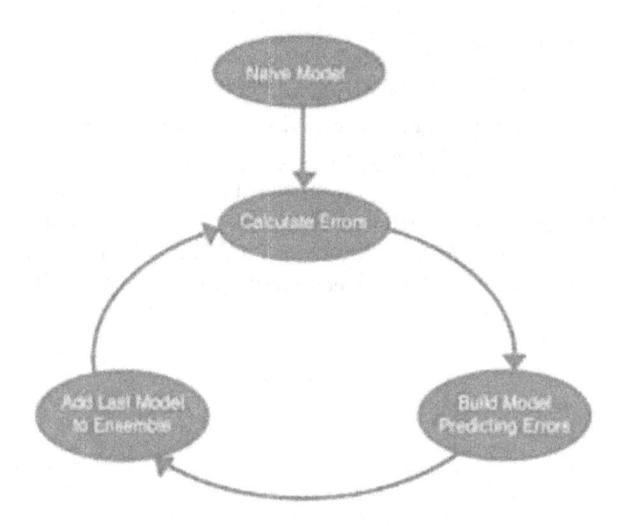

FIGURE 11.6 XGBoost of Boosted Trees [13].

11.2.7 Extra Trees

The Extra-Tree method was given with the main focus of further sampling tree building in the background of the numerical input type ,where the best cut-point is accountable for a large quantity of the inconsistency of the induced tree. The Extra Trees algorithm works by designing a huge number of decision trees from the exercise dataset. Projections are given by averaging the forecast of the decision trees in deterioration.

11.3 RELATED WORK

Lertworaprachaya designed a model for creating membership values using decision trees. Decision trees consider only fuzzy membership type values [9–11]. So, the author uses membership values for making a model and employs tree induction methods for effective results. The authors also determined the specific values and give effective results using fuzzy sets. There are many examples of how to make an effective approach. Bahnsen designed a cost-sensitive algorithm with decision tree parameters. With different databases, from applications like credit card fraud detection, the author gives their effective method. Blanco designed the other pattern that performs combined actions with a different approach [12–16]. In this pattern, parameter changes by changing the structure of the tree, which gives the comparative change in outputs. Then, Blanco gives another model for replacing the main tree and improves the result of the model. An effective model is also viewed as classifiers, and assumptions of models are used for deterministic results [17–20]. This pattern is related to algorithms based on the decision tree for drift selection criteria. The author shows that their effective pattern gives valuable outcomes with different flow chart structures so that they can maintain the time boundary conditions and the number of samples used [21, 22].

11.4 PROPOSED WORK

In this hybrid structure, a combination of XGBoost, Extra trees and Gaussian Classifier is used, as shown in Figure 11.7. First, Parkinson's disease dataset is used from the UCI library. After pre-processing the data splits the input and output pulses and initializes the XGBoost, Extra trees and Gaussian Classifier for train test splits. Their train pulses are verified with test pulses. Then the data is standardized by reducing the column size and extracting important features with 221 columns. Then train the test splits, use extra tree classifier to calculate the Gini index from

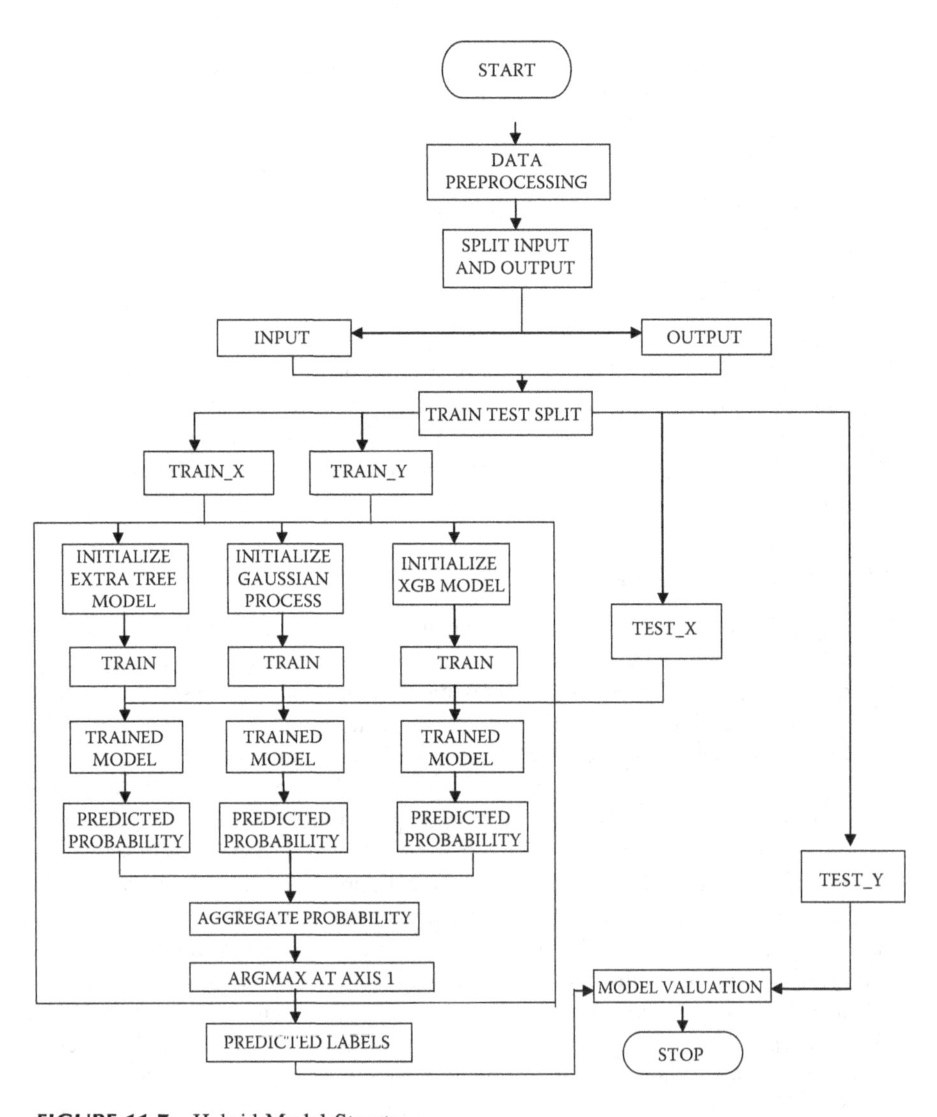

FIGURE 11.7 Hybrid Model Structure.

random feature with respect to target and find out the maximum depth specification to create the split of features with highest Gini index as shown in Figure 11.8 and Table 11.1. Repeat the steps for different samples of data and create n estimator trees to reduce the error of the previous tree, as shown in Figure 11.9. Then apply Gaussian process classification training and calculate the parameters of conditional probability. Apply the Argmax on axis 1 to get predicted labels. After reducing the column size, apply the hybrid structure and find out the aggregate predicted probability parameters for each class to compare the predicted values with actual ones to find out the results and evaluate the model.

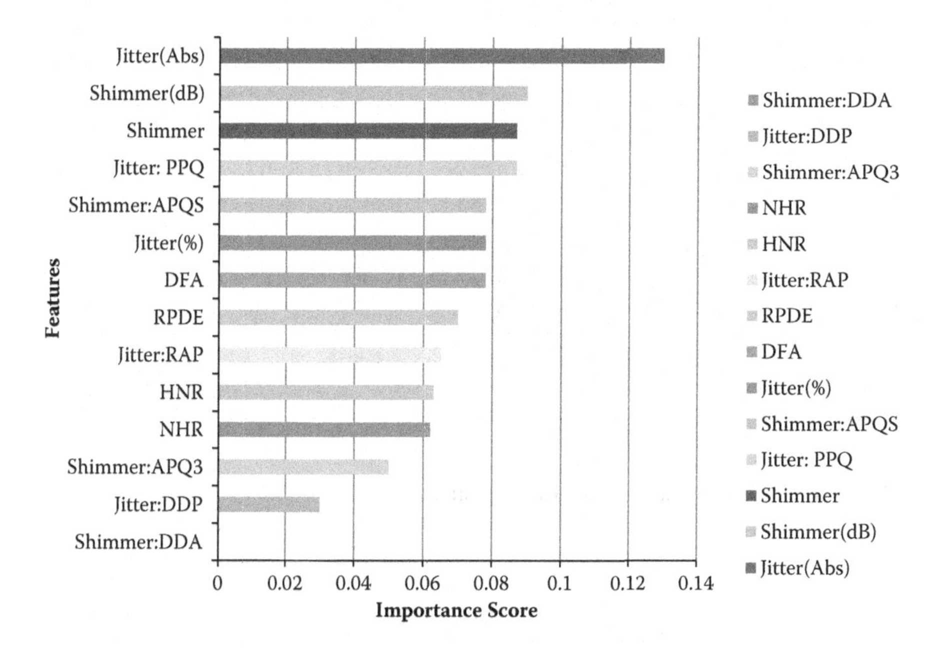

FIGURE 11.8 Important Features with Their Score Level.

TABLE 11.1
Important Features Value

	Jitter(Abs)	Shimmer(dB)	Shimmer	Jitter:PPQ
0	1.702385	−0.303385	−0.379977	1.816570
1	2.059402	0.229104	0.038264	2.475958
2	2.416418	−0.154288	−0.175847	2.870662
3	2.416418	−0.061102	−0.114299	2.485245
4	3.130451	0.117281	0.107416	3.460395

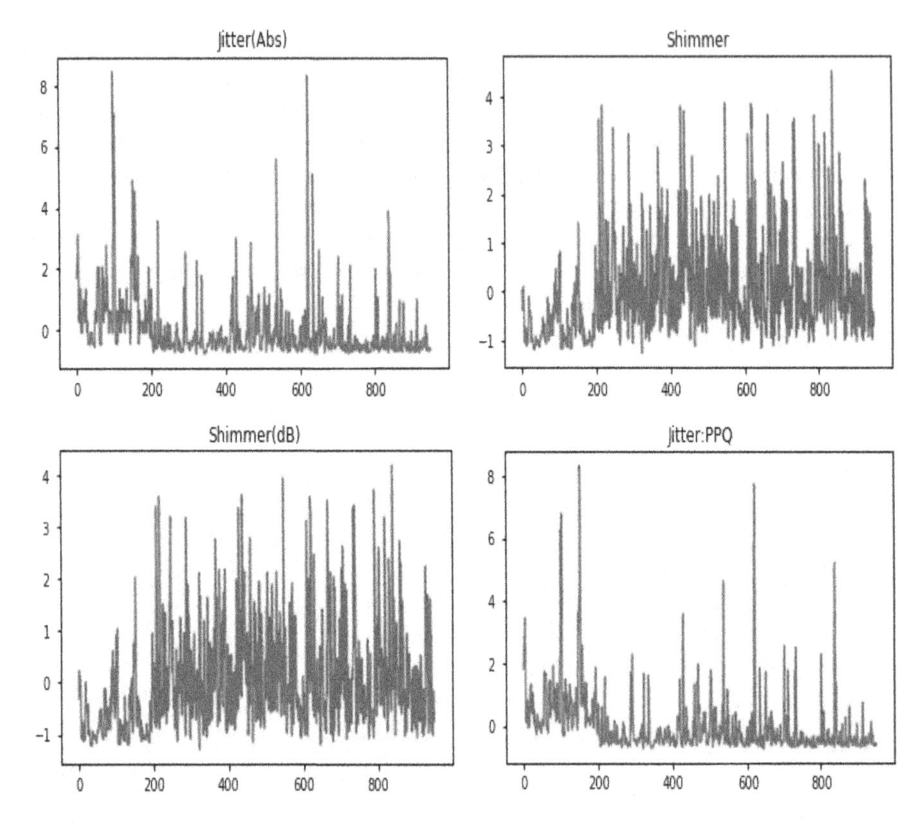

FIGURE 11.9 Important Feature Concentrations.

These parameters are:

- Jitter(Abs): is used in frequency for determining the time to time variation.
- Jitter: DDP: is the average of contrast among jitter pattern.
- Shimmer: is displayed in a percentage and it is the ratio of consecutive period amplitude to the average amplitude.
- Shimmer: DDA: Changes in average amplitudes of periods.

11.5 RESULTS AND DISCUSSIONS

This hybrid model results in a high accuracy level 77.62% in comparison to the other classifiers as the hybrid is a combination of various classifiers with their best feature and concentration value for giving the best result and accuracy level, as shown in Figure 11.10. This result is based on the four selected parameters of Parkinson's disease by using various column reducing algorithms. This model is a combination of XGBoost, Extra trees and Gaussian Classifier. First, find out their train pulses from their trained model and evaluate their conditional probabilities. Then the average aggregate of these probabilities is marked with label structure and

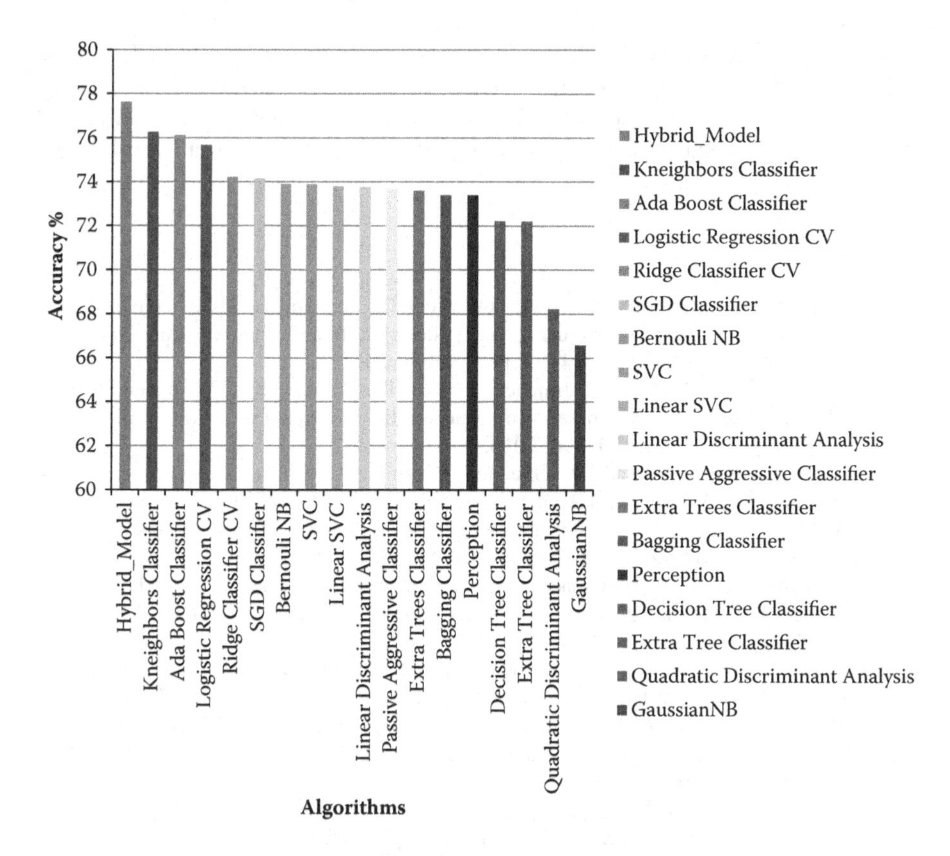

FIGURE 11.10 Hybrid Model Results.

examined with other classifier like Kneighbour, Adaboost, Logistic regression, Support vector and linear support vector. By using this model, we can easily detect the speech impairment level of humans and use effective techniques for communicating with each other. The tests have been carried out over the Parkinson's dataset and we selected the four parameters using specific parameter selection methods. After reducing the column size, it is necessary to apply the hybrid structure and find out the aggregate predicted probability parameters for each class to compare the predicted values with actual to find out the results and evaluate the model. All analyses are performed on a wide dataset obtained from the UCI library.

11.6 CONCLUSION

This paper presented a hybrid model structure that gives comparative results with various speech recognition classification algorithms. Classification is an effective method to detect new parameters depending on the output received from previous training set parameters. For effective machine learning results, it uses a specific model, effective techniques, knowledge parameters and advanced trees algorithm for displaying the valuable results. A hybrid structure algorithm needs a little amount of dataset information to estimate the mandatory parameters so that an effective result can be displayed. We have selected the top four speech-related parameters and obtained a higher accuracy level of 77.62% with a hybrid model compared to the other classifiers.

REFERENCES

1. Crockett, A. Latham, N. Whitton, "On predicting learning styles in conversational intelligent tutoring systems using fuzzy decision trees," *International Journal of Human-Computer Studies*, vol. 97, pp. 98–115, 2017.
2. F. Blanco, J. C. Ávila, G. R. Jiménez, A. Carvalho, A.O. Díaz, R. M. Bueno, "Online adaptive decision trees based on concentration inequalities," *Knowledge-Based Systems*, vol. 104, pp. 179–194, 2016.
3. A. C. Bahnsen, D. Aouada, B. Ottersten, "Example dependent cost-sensitive decision trees," *Expert Systems with Applications*, vol. 42, pp. 6609–6619, 2015.
4. X. Pan, Y. Luo, Y. Xu, "K-nearest neighbour based structural twin support vector machine," *Knowledge Based Systems*, vol. 88, pp. 34–44, 2015.
5. Mandal,I., Sairam,N. New machine learning algorithms for prediction of Parkinson's disease *International Journal of Systems Science*, 45(3), pp. 647–666, 2014. DOI: 0.1080/00207721.2012.724114.
6. Y. Lertworaprachaya, Y. Yang, R. John, "Interval-valued fuzzy decision trees with optimal neighbourhood perimeter," *Applied Soft Computing*, vol. 24, pp. 851– 866, 2014.
7. Mandal, I., and Sairam, N. Accurate prediction of coronary artery disease using reliable diagnosis system *Journal of Medical Systems*, vol. 36 (5), Pages 3353–3373, 2012. DOI: 10.1007/s10916-012-9828-0.
8. Mandal, I., Sairam, N. Enhanced classification performance using computational intelligence *Communications in Computer and Information Science, 204CCIS*, vol. 204, pp. 384–391, 2011. DOI: 10.1007/978-3-642-24043-0_39.
9. Yu, Zhiwen, Peinan Luo, Jane You, Hau-San Wong, Hareton Leung, Si Wu, Jun Zhang, and Guoqiang Han "Incremental semi-supervised clustering ensemble for high dimensional data clustering." *IEEE Transactions on Knowledge and Data Engineering, vol.* 28(3),701–714, 2015.
10. Patil, Harsh Kupwade, and Ravi Seshadri. "Big data security and privacy issues in healthcare." *In 2014 IEEE International Congress on Big Data*, pp. 762–765. IEEE, 2014.
11. Rohit Raja, Tilendra Shishir Sinha, Ravi Prakash Dubey, Recognition of human-face from side-view using progressive switching pattern and soft-computing technique, *Association for the Advancement of Modelling and Simulation Techniques in Enterprises, Advance B*, vol. 58(1), pp. 14–34, 2015, ISSN: -1240-4543.
12. T. Chen, H. Li, Q. Yang, and Y. Yu. General functional matrix factorization using gradient boosting. In Proceeding of 30th *International Conference on Machine Learning (ICML'13)*, vol. 1, pages 436–444, 2013.
13. Himalaya Gohiya, Harsh Lohiya and Kailash Patidar, *A Survey of XGBoost System in International Journal of Advanced Technology & Engineering Research (IJATER)*, vol. 8(3), May 2018. A Survey: Tree Boosting System Page range 12–17.
14. Aaditya Jain," Text classification by combining text classifiers to improve the efficiency of classification", *International Journal of Computer Application*, ISSN: 2250-1797, vol. 6, March- April 2016: 126–129.
15. R. Jothikumar, R.V. Sivabalan, "Analysis of classification algorithms for heart disease prediction and its accuracies," *Middle-East Journal of Scientific Research 24 (Recent Innovations in Engineering, Technology, Management & Applications)* 24: 200–206, 2016.

16. T. Sharma, A. Sharma, V. Mansotra, "Performance analysis of data mining classification techniques on public health care data," *International Journal of Innovative Research in Computer and Communication Engineering*, vol. 4(6), June 2016. 11381–11386.
17. S. Sharma, V. Sharma, A. Sharma, "Performance based evaluation of various machine learning classification techniques for chronic kidney disease diagnosis". *International Journal of Modern Computer Science (IJMCS) ISSN: 2320-7868 (Online)*, vol. 4(3), June, 2016.
18. E. Venkatesan, T. Velmurugan, "Performance analysis of decision tree algorithms for breast cancer classification," *Indian Journal of Science and Technology*, Vol 8(29), DOI: 10.17485/ijst/2015/v8i29/84646, November 20151–8.
19. E. Nafise, A. Farshad, Wavelet adaptation for automatic voice disorders sorting. *Computers in Biology and Medicine* 43, 699–704, 2013.
20. Rohit Raja, Tilendra Shishir Sinha, Ravi Prakash Dubey, Soft computing and LGXP techniques for ear authentication using progressive switching pattern, Published in *International Journal of Engineering and Future Technology*, vol. 2(2), pp. 66–86, 2016, ISSN: 2455-6432.
21. Aaditya Desai, Dr. Sunil Rai, "Analysis of machine learning algorithms using WEKA" *International Conference & Workshop on Recent Trends in Technology*, (TCET) 2012.
22. Xu, X., Yang, G. Robust manifold classification based on semi supervised learning *International Journal of Advancements in Computing Technology*, 5(8), pp. 174–183, 2013. DOI: 10.4156/ijact.vol5.issue6.21.

12 Advanced Ensemble Machine Learning Model for Balanced BioAssays

Lokesh Pawar, Anuj Kumar Sharma, Dinesh Kumar, and Rohit Bajaj

CONTENTS

12.1 INTRODUCTION

ML is a technique by which a model can learn from the training dataset. Machine Learning is one of the common forms of Artificial Intelligence (AI); According to the report by the global research and advisory firm, *Gartner*, Artificial Intelligence is expected to generate jobs close to 2.3 million by the year 2020 [1]. Machine Learning is a statistical approach to handle the dataset and to apply different algorithms to predict the results for the testing dataset. Machine learning in the medical field has recently achieved greater heights. Recently, Google has worked on a Machine Learning algorithm to identify cancer and tumor patients [2]. Many other universities and organizations are using the Deep Learning algorithm to classify skin cancer [3, 4].

The report *International Research View* reported in 2018 that the global medical discovery market was estimated at nearly $0.7 billion in 2016 nearly and was expected to progress at the Compound Annual Growth Rate of 12.6% in this decade. Artificial Intelligence and Machine Learning (ML) is encouraging many researchers to find inexpensive solutions in numerous fields such as medical discovery and the like. By the end of this decade, Artificial Intelligence will have the capability to save $0.07 billion in the medical field. In this Research paper, there is a work with the Biopsy Dataset consisting of 144 attributes based on which will be applied on different classifiers, and then after choosing the Best 10 out of all the classifiers based on their accuracy, we will ensemble the classifiers using Stacking and Voting to attain more accuracy. We'll be using WEKA to create the ensemble model [5, 6].

The biopsy could be a diagnostic assay which will be a procedure to obviate a bit of tissue or a sample of cells from the body to be analyzed during a laboratory. If an individual is experiencing signs and symptoms, or if the doctor has discovered an area of concern, a diagnostic assay may be ordered to figure out whether or not cancer is present or it is due to another condition [7]. While imaging tests, like X-rays, square measure useful in detective work lots or areas of abnormality, they alone cannot differentiate cancerous cells from noncancerous cells. For the bulk of cancers, the sole thanks to building a definitive designation are to perform a diagnostic test to gather cells for closer examination.

Every year, pathologists diagnose 14 million new patients with cancer around the world. These millions of individuals will face years of uncertainty. Pathologists have been diagnosing cancer diagnoses and prognoses for many years. Most pathologists have a 96–98% success rate for the designation of cancer. On their part, they are highly capable. The problem comes with the other part. The prognosis is that part of a biopsy that comes when cancer has been diagnosed; it predicts the course of the illness. It is time for a number of successive steps to be taken in pathology [8]. ML has key advantages over pathologists. Firstly, machines will work a lot quicker than humans. A Biopsy test typically takes a diagnostician ten days ,whereas a computer will do thousands of biopsies during a matter of seconds.

Machines will do one thing that humans aren't that good at. They'll repeat themselves thousands of times without becoming exhausted. After each iteration, the machine repeats the method to try and do it higher. Humans can work hard to make the result perfect but they still cannot match the computational power of the computer.

12.2 RELATED WORK

In this research paper firstly the supervised dataset of biopsy is taken from the Internet and the class is balanced using the Class Balancer in WEKA. There are weka filters supervised; for instance Class Balancer, a straightforward filter that gives instance weights that every category of instances can have identical weight and also the total add of instance weights within the dataset remains the same [9].

When weka classifier meta Filtered Classifier is used with this filter and also the base classifier doesn't execute Weighted Instances Handler then the weights can once more be wont to kind a likelihood distribution for sampling with replacement. This can yield a training set wherever each class is (approximately) balanced. And after applying the *Class Balancer,* different classifiers are applied to the dataset and then the author prepared the graphs for their Accuracy, True Positive Rate, False Positive Rate, and ROC [10].

The Classifiers that are used in work are Random Forest, Random Tree, REPTree, Decision Stump, Decision Table, PART, ZeroR, JRip, Input Mapped Classifier, AdaBoost M1, Bagging, LogitBoost, Random Subspace, Multi Class Classifier Updateable, Randomizable Filtered Classifier, Ibk, LWL, Logistics, Multilayer Perceptron, SGDText, Simple Logistics, SMO, Bayes Net, Naive Bayes, Naive Bayes, Multinomial Text, Naive Bayes Updateable, Filtered Classifier, Multi Class Classifier, Random Committee, J48. The best 10 classifiers were chosen based on their Accuracy, True Positive Rate, False Positive Rate, and ROC. Table 1.1 below shows the performance of the chosen classifiers. By implementing this proposed advanced model using ensembling, those samples which were having meager outcome will now have high balance accuracy [11].

12.3 PROPOSED WORK

The dataset is given to the Machine Learning Model i.e., Weka. The classes are balanced using class balancer i.e., weka, filters, supervised, instances. Class balancer and selective instances are auto-fetched. As already discussed, various classifiers are tested on the dataset, and corresponding Accuracy, True Positive Rate, FP Rate, and ROC are recorded and the top 10 classifiers are selected since the results are not very precise. Therefore, for more accuracy and precision, the ensemble model is required. The author employed STACKING and VOTING to acquire more accuracy in biopsy results. A simple Logistics ensembled-based machine took the lead and comes out to be the Advanced Model.

12.3.1 Ensemble Classification

The ML model is developed to predict the active as well as inactive bioassay compound. To handle it 10 different models are used; namely, Random Subspace, J48, SMO, Bagging, Simple Logistics, LWL, Multiclass Classifier Updateable, Ibk, Naive Bayes and Naive Bayes Updateable. The Bayes Net classifier is linked to the Direct Acyclic Graph whose knobs correspond to variables in the Bayes Net sensitivity. Navie Bayes Classifier is designed for use in the supervised induction task. This classifier is based on the cluster of the classification algorithms derived from Bayes' Theorem. It can also be seen as the specialized form of the Bayesian Network. It assumes that the predictive result is independent of the given attributes. It is assumed that each attribute or feature contribute equally to predict the result. The motive of the Navie Bayes Classifier is to precisely calculate the class of testing attributes from the training attributes include the class information. The Sequential minimal optimization is a classifier used for solving the quadratic programming dilemma that arises during the training of SVM. J48 labeled the data and based on that data, it represents a choice tree that's used for classification.

12.4 EXPERIMENTAL INVESTIGATION

The Figure 12.1 shows the Dataset and the experimental setup of the model.

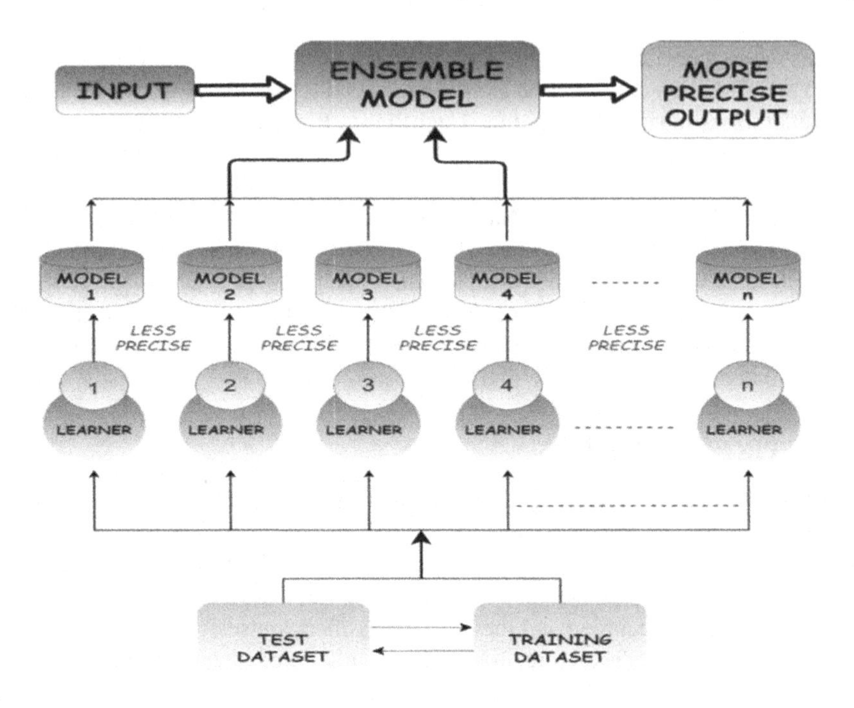

FIGURE 12.1 Abstract View.

12.4.1 Dataset Report

A total of 15 Datasets were formed using examining and testing so a decision can be made. Every dataset has 15 training and 15 testing subsets in Database. There are two parts of the full dataset, primary and confirmatory that has five datasets are of primary screening and eight datasets are of an area of substantiating screening. There are also two datasets for each primary and confirmatory screening, which primary screening of bioassay permit examining and testing so a decision can be made of binding measure of tiny compounds while not classifying it. One of the problems of using the bioassay data is that the data is not curated and is potentially erroneous. However, there is no search facility to retrieve the Primary Screening results together with its corresponding Confirmatory Screen (if there is one). Finding corresponding confirmatory bioassays is only achieved by manually going through each primary screen webpage and seeing if there is one in the related bioassays section. The problem is complicated further as sometimes several primary screen bioassay data is used for the one confirmatory screen and vice versa. However, there is a lack of publicly-available bioassay data due to the fact that most HTS technology is held at private commercial organisations. On the other hand, mistakes occur throughout the primary High Throughput Screening method for that secondary screening performs on the primary screening data. It is planned to confirm successes ability by a series of supportive assays. The main purpose of secondary screening is to spot the helpful response of composites somewhat, making it a high throughput format. In this study, the primary dataset is taken to estimate biopsy. The total compounds are 4279 with 144 options of

3423 of various medical instances in the dataset. The parameters embrace dual options that facilitate the total calculation of active and inactive medicine.

12.4.2 Experimental Setting

In this research, different models were created using the WEKA Software and the Classifiers of WEKA are also used. This research aims to measure the Accuracy, TP Measure, FP Measure, ROC and make predictions of the classifiers. And after that creating ensemble models to increase the calculated factors i.e., Accuracy, TP Measure, FP Measure, ROC of the classifiers. The training and testing dataset are two forms of the dataset.

12.5 RESULTS

The following section discusses the results and assessment of the proposed advanced model on the dataset.

12.5.1 Assessment of Results

The assessment of the proposed model is performed using parameters like Accuracy, True Positive Rate, False Positive Rate, F-Measure, MCC, and ROC as shown in Table 12.1. It describes the assessment of all the classifiers i.e., Random Subspace, J48, SMO, Bagging, Simple Logistics, LWL, Multiclass Classifier Updateable, Ibk, Naive Bayes and Naive Bayes Updateable and Advanced Simple Logistics. In Figure 12.2 graphs are plotted based on Table 12.1 to show the assessment of diverse classifiers. Figure 12.2.a describes the accuracy of the different classifiers and it shows the Advanced Simple Logistics has the best accuracy between the classifiers, as it is an ensemble model.

Figure 12.2.b describes ROC curve that shows how classifiers are behaving normally. It also draws the true positive rate adjacent to the false positive rate. So, a higher positive rate provides the best result. That, Advanced Simple Logistics is the best ROC in comparison to other classifiers. Figure 12.2.c describes True Positive Rate, Naive Bayes, and Simple Logistics perform well to categorize the instances correctly because Naive Bayes and Simple Logistics both are ensembled algorithms. Figure 12.2.d describes the False Positive Rate, which shows falsely classified instances. Random Subspace performs best to falsely classify the instances with others.

12.5.2 Assessment of the Model on the Dataset

Current section assesses the assessment of the proposed advanced ensemble on the dataset. The results are presented in Table 12.2. The parameters are True Positive Rate, False Positive Rate, Precision, and Accuracy. A comparison of these parameters of the proposed model has been done with the previous research results on the same dataset. Previous, the work has implemented RS, J48, SMO, Bagging, Simple Logistics, LWL, Multiclass Classifier Updateable, Ibk, Naive Bayes, and Naive Bayes Updateable for the proposed model.

TABLE 12.1
Performance of All the Classifiers

Classifiers	Random Sub Space	J48	SMO	Bagging	Simple Logistics	LWL	Multiclass Classifier Updateable	Ibk	Naive Bayes	Naive Bayes Updateable	Advanced Simple Logistics
Accuracy	59.48	61.20	61.32	61.61	61.87	61.97	65.36	66.07	**70.50**	**70.50**	**73.5387**
True Positive Rate	0.595	0.612	0.613	0.616	0.619	0.620	0.654	0.661	0.705	0.705	**0.735**
False Positive Rate	0.405	0.388	0.387	0.384	0.381	0.380	0.346	0.339	0.295	0.295	0.265
F-Measure	0.540	0.553	0.554	0.557	0.585	0.614	0.614	0.620	0.692	0.692	0.729
MCC	0.262	0.325	0.329	0.341	0.289	0.247	0.400	0.425	0.490	0.449	0.494
ROC	0.626	0.613	0.613	0.737	0.647	0.556	0.654	0.710	0.655	0.655	**0.737**

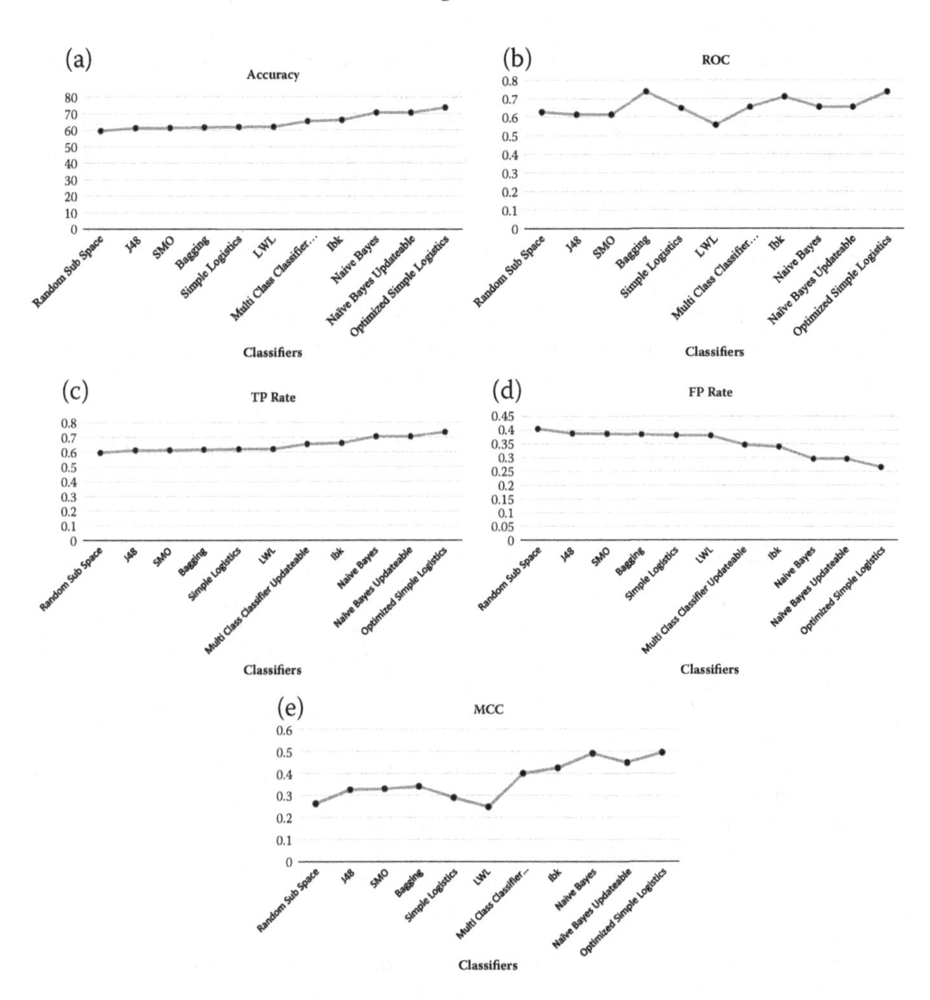

FIGURE 12.2 Assessment Charts of Accuracy, ROC, True Positive Rate, False Positive Rate, and MCC with Classifiers.

TABLE 12.2
Results of Assessment of the Proposed Advanced Ensemble on the Dataset

Classifiers	Random Sub Space	SMO	LWL	Naive Bayes	Advanced Simple Logistics
Accuracy	59.48	61.32	61.97	70.50	**73.5387**
True Positive Rate	0.595	0.613	0.620	0.705	**0.735**
FP Rate	0.405	0.387	0.380	0.295	0.265
Precision	0.681	0.739	0.627	0.746	0.759

The best accuracy of 70.4976% has been calculated by the Naive Bayes and Naive Bayes Updatable algorithm. On the contrary, after ensembling, Advanced Simple Logistics gave an accuracy of **73.5387%** only. It has been observed that after ensembling the accuracy of the model has achieved higher accuracy and predictive performance in comparison to previous models.

12.6 CONCLUSION

Machine Learning has been evolving in every nook and corner. The results are not only automated but more humanly and rapidly. Just as the authors advanced the classifiers for the results of Biopsy, such optimization techniques can be employed in different scenarios as well. Ensemble is amongst the best optimization techniques to achieve more accurate results. The existing classifiers can be ensembled together to acquire more precision.

REFERENCES

1. Luengo, J., Fernández, A., García, S., Herrera, F. (2011). Addressing data complexity for imbalanced data sets: analysis of SMOTE-based oversampling and evolutionary under sampling. *Soft Computing*, 15(10): 1909–1936. https://doi.org/10.1007/s00500-010-0625-8.
2. Chen, B., Wild, D.J. (2010). PubChem BioAssays as a data source for predictive models. *Journal of Molecular Graphics and Modelling*, 28(5): 420–426. https://doi.org/10.1016/j.jmgm.2009.10.001.
3. Russo, D.P., Strickland, J., Karmaus, A.L., Wang, W., Shende, S., Hartung, T., Aleksunes, L.M., Zhu, H. (2019). Nonanimal models for acute toxicity evaluations: applying data-driven profiling and read-across. *Environmental Health Perspectives*, 127(4): 047001. https://doi.org/10.1289/EHP3614.
4. Kotsiantis, S.B., Zaharakis, I.D., Pintelas, P.E. (2006). Machine learning: a review of classification and combining techniques. *Artificial Intelligence Review*, 26(3): 159–190. https://doi.org/10.1007/s10462-007-9052-3.
5. Platt, J.C. (1998). Sequential minimal optimization: *A fast algorithm for training support vector machines*. ISBN: 0-262-19416-3, 185–208.
6. Belgiu, M., Drăguţ, L. (2016). Random forest in remote sensing: a review of applications and future directions. *ISPRS Journal of Photogrammetry and Remote Sensing*, 24-31.
7. Wang, Y., Xiao, J., Suzek, T.O., Zhang, J., Wang, J., Zhou, Z.G., Han, L.Y., Karapetyan, K., Dracheva, S., Shoemaker, B.A., Bolton, E., Gindulyte, A., Bryant, S.H. (2011). PubChem's BioAssay database. *Nucleic Acids Research*, 40(D1): D400–D412. https://doi.org/10.1093/nar/gkr1132.
8. Stork, C., Wagner, J., Friedrich, N.O., de Bruyn Kops, C., Šícho, M., Kirchmair, J. (2018). Hit dexter: a machine-learning model for the prediction of frequent hitters. *ChemMedChem*, 13(6): 564–571. https://doi.org/10.1002/cmdc.201700673.
9. Niculescu, M.S. (2017). Optical method for improving the accuracy of biochemical assays. *In 2017 E-Health and Bioengineering Conference (EHB)*, pp. 381–385. https://doi.org/10.1109/EHB.2017.7995441.
10. Nielsen, T.D., Jensen, F.V. Bayesian networks, and decision graphs. *Springer Science & Business Media*. accessed on 4 June 2009.
11. Laxmikant Tiwari, Rohit Raja, Vaibhav Sharma, Rohit Miri (2019), Adaptive neuro fuzzy inference system based fusion of medical image, *International Journal of Research in Electronics and Computer Engineering*, 7(2), pp. 2086–2091, ISSN: 2393-9028 (PRINT) |ISSN: 2348-2281.

13 Lung Segmentation and Nodule Detection in 3D Medical Images Using Convolution Neural Network

Rohit Raja, Sandeep Kumar, Shilpa Rani, and K. Ramya Laxmi

CONTENTS

13.1 INTRODUCTION

Lungs are the most important organs for our cellular respiration system which is situated in the chest cavity. Lungs are a set of spongy organs which allow us to breathe properly. Lungs are responsible for providing oxygen to the human body and also expel carbon dioxide from the body. The exchange of these gases is called respiration. In today's lifestyle lung cancer is a common disease and it's also a reason of a greater number of deaths around the world. Lung cancer is a deadly cancer other than breast cancer, bone cancer etc. Smoking is a common cause of lung cancer but people who don't have smoking habits can also get lung cancer. However, chances are ten times less for a nonsmoker than for a person who smokes. Diagnosing the lung tumor at an early stage is a very difficult task. Yet if it is detected in the last stage, the only option is to remove the cancerous lung. Therefore, it is necessary that it should be detected in the early stage or first stage of the cancer.There are different ways of detecting the cancerous tumor such as CT scan, MRI, PET and so on etc[1].

Three-dimensional (3D) [2, 3] advanced pictures were typically procured by scanners likewise Computed Tomography (CT) framework, Magnetic Resonance Imaging (MRI) framework, Positron Emission Tomography (PET) framework, Ultra Sound Imaging (USI) framework, 3D optical/3D electron magnifying instrument, 3D confocal magnifying instrument, Range Image Sensor (RIS) framework, Synthetic Aperture Radar (SAR), Scanning Ground Penetrating Radar (SGPR) [4,5]. The 3D computerized picture information obtained utilizing such scanners are basically the trademark impressions of different parts under the checking zone of explicit intrigue. One won't have the option to envision the shrouded pieces of a 3D picture so as to make significant translations. In this way, handling the 3D picture information is about the abstraction of bodily, morphological and auxiliary belongings of concealed pieces of the picture. For example, a Magnetic Resonance Imaging is handled to extricate concealed subtleties, for the most part visual in nature.

Exact insights concerning the shrouded parts could be acquired just when preparation strategies are dependable and vigorous. Malignant growth of the lung is brought about by sporadic development of cells in lung tissue due to smoking. It very well may be treated by recognizing it early. Screening can be actualized to distinguish knobs. Knob is clarified as a white spot present on the lungs which can be seen on X-beam and CT filter pictures [6]. Knobs is of 2 sorts:

1. Begin knob (if a knob is 3 cm is called as start knob)
2. Lung mass (this knob is bigger than 3 cm is called as lung mass)

It should be dispensed in as timely a manner as could be expected under the circumstances. Lung knobs might not have any connection with other knobs. It is basic to ascertain the knob size cautiously to clarify the harm factor [7]. Pictures from CT and X-beam can be taken to distinguish the size of knob. It has been tried with LDCT sweep to recognize lung malignancy. Computer aided design frameworks are utilized to recognize reasons of enthusiasm for the image that gives data. In regard to harm there are two sorts: CADe (PC supported location framework) and CADX (computer-aided diagnosis). We can distinguish and give data and movement of knobs by utilizing above CADX and CADe. These assist in curtailing endless CT examination reports [8].

Malignant lung growth is the most well-known disease dependent on the flow insights of frequency and death rate. Computer-aided detection (CADe) framework has been intended to assist the radiologist/master to improve the exactness and viability in the discovery of malignant lung growth. In the current work a CADe framework is used to portion the lung area and distinguish knobs from CT Scan

Image utilizing Convolution Neural Network. The lung Computed Tomography checks are obtained from Lungs picture Data bank Group - Image Database Resource Initiative database [8, 9]. The proposed study consists of four phases:

i. Separation of lung parenchyma via Fuzzy-c-implies bunching calculation,
ii. Nodule extraction utilizing a Gober Filter Method,
iii. Noise evacuation utilizing CCAbased methodology, and
iv. Finding of lungs knob by Extracted include by CNN.

The outcomes were approved beside the clarified ground reality given by four master radiologists. The proposed investigation fundamentally lessens the quantity of bogus positives (FPs) in the distinguished knob applicants. This strategy shows a general exactness of over 80% at a diminished FPs/examine pace of 0.50. The proposed framework demonstrated an improvement in lung knob location precision and can be usable in clinical settings [10, 11].

13.2 REVIEW OF LITERATURE

Various writings propose that lung disease has become a common condition, a significant challenge to eradicate or treat, and one of the main sources of death, particularly in developing nations. The findings include identification of lung knob precisely is the region of center for the specialists doing innovative work exercises. Normally, small injuries cannot be provided the assistance of X-beams; and, accordingly, figured tomography (CT) is utilized for the location of malignant lung growth. An enormous number of cases; less survey time; the strength of the techniques for location are among many of the significant difficulties in the field of lung malignancy finding (Sinha, G.R., Patil, S., 2014). PC helped conclusion (CAD) based strategies be utilized in all cutting-edge examination and finding research centers. Bogus ID of dangerous components is a typical source of confusion in manual identification of the disease [Patil, D. S. what's more, Kuchanur, M., 2012]. The computerized approach is created in CAD, wherein some picture preparing apparatuses are additionally utilized in prehandling; highlight extraction; and post-handling of the clinical pictures. Scarcely any exploration papers on CAD exist but those that do [Chaudhary A. what's more, Singh, S. S., 2012], [Hadavi, N., Nordin, M., Shojaeipour A., 2014] stress building a productive and precise robotized approach for malignant lung growth identification. We have actualized lung disease discovery utilizing fluffy derivation framework (FIS) to recognize the conspicuous destructive cells, including every one of the four phases of CAD-like other examination work. Fluffy induction rules were applied to get precise outcomes for lung malignancy location.

Camarlinghi, N (2012), use CAD procedure for recognizing aspiratory knobs in CT checks. Abdullah A. A. what's more, Shaharum, S. M. (2013) use feed forward neural system to group lung knobs in X-Ray pictures; though with just few highlights; for example, territory, edge and shape. The suitable arrangement of highlights and grouping strategies came about due to the helpless exactness of CAD-based conclusion results. Kuruvilla, J. furthermore, Gunavathi, K. (2014)

consider six particular boundaries, including skewness, fifth and 6th central minutes extricated from sectioned single cuts featuring the highlights as proposed in (Abdullah A. A. what's more, Shaharum, S. M., 2013). The feed forward back engendering neural system is prepared to assess exactness for various highlights independently. Bellotti, R., et al. (2017) present another PC helped discovery framework for knob location utilizing dynamic form based model in CT pictures. This work guarantees a high location pace of 88.5% with a normal of 6.6 bogus positives (FPs) per CT check on 15 CT filters, yet the size of database was not huge. Hayashibe, R. (1996), execute a programmed strategy on mass chest radiographs for discovery of new lung knobs. Kanazawa, K. (1996) removes highlights and examinations of the lung and pneumonic vein locales and afterward uses characterized rules to perform analysis, which was utilized in the identification of tumor up-and-comers from helical CT pictures.

In (Kumar, A., Kumar, P., 2006) marker-driven watershed division separates seeds that show the nearness of articles or foundation at explicit picture areas. The marker areas are considered as local minima and afterward the watershed calculation is applied. Mori et al, (1996) do extraction of bronchus region from 3D chest X-beam CT pictures. Starting finding of division of CT check utilizing convolution neural system (CNN) grouping, was featured (Sandeep A. Dwivedi, R., Borse, B., Yametkar, 2014). Alawaa, W., Mahammad, N., Badr, A. (2017) [12–14] suggests new technique for effective preparing and recognition of malignant components found in lung CT pictures. Current writing proposes that there is a lot of work that has been now done in the field of malignant lung growth recognition. Be that as it may, the exactness has not been endeavored to improve with the assistance of fluffy based methodologies.

The CAD framework is in present day a mainstream which is taken as a second opinion for radiologists in the field of lung malignancy recognition. Computer aided design framework is fundamentally the total bundle which contains Computer aided-detection(CADe) and computer-aided diagnosis (CADx).

13.3 RATIONALE OF THE STUDY

In Detection of Nodule and Lung Segmentation numerous computer-aided diagnostic structures had been intended to assist the radiologist. The two fundamental factors which influence the exactness and accuracy in discovery of malignant lung growth are particularly that knob who has comparable power and they are associated with a vessel and the knob with normal feeble edges, thus it is hard to characterize the limits. In the current work the fundamental target is to deal with the two above issues by CADe framework for division and recognition of knobs structure with CT Scan Images utilizing CNN strategy and Morphological Image preparing. The upside of utilizing CNN for a broad list of capabilities like surface complexity, connection and shape are extricated. The current work has been breaking down utilizing the information of various subjects of a range of ages to help bring down the quantity of exclusions and to diminish the time expected to inspect the sweep by a radiologist. There are five issues that can be related with CADs for malignant lung growth discovery. The principal issue is the discovery of clamors and misfortune less data in the CT picture. Because of quality of clamor, the exhibition of the framework may corrupt. Therefore, it must be evacuated and consequently packed, for getting better outcomes during acknowledgment process. The subsequent issue is to identify the limits or shapes of the pictures coming about to lung division of the CT picture. Figure 13.1 shows morphological preparing on picture "X" alongside organizing component "Z". There are numerous methods are available for the detection of lung tumor and most of the methods use the basic steps for the detection of tumor. Steps of tumor detection is represented in Figure 13.2.

13.3.1 Morphological Processing of the Digital Image

Numerical morphologies are significant worldview utilized in picture investigation and instrument vision application. These parts give an outline of numerical morphology as a way to deal with shallow identity and volumetric highlights in 3D computerized pictures. It likewise characterizes certain fundamental morphological tasks of widening and disintegration on 2D and 3D pictures [15, 16].

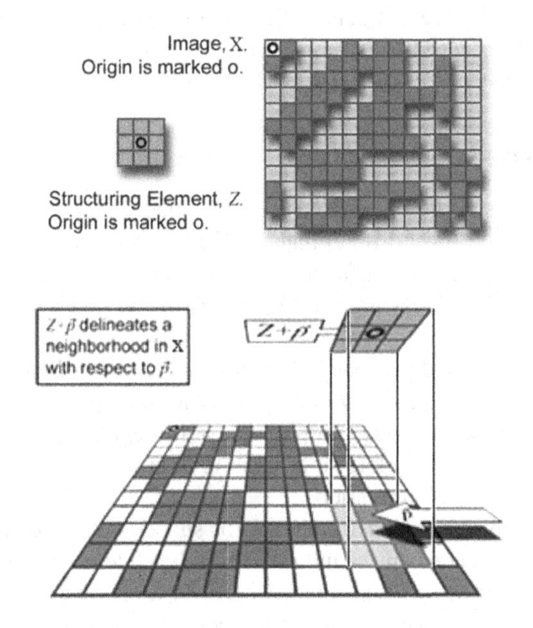

FIGURE 13.1 Structuring Element's Processing.

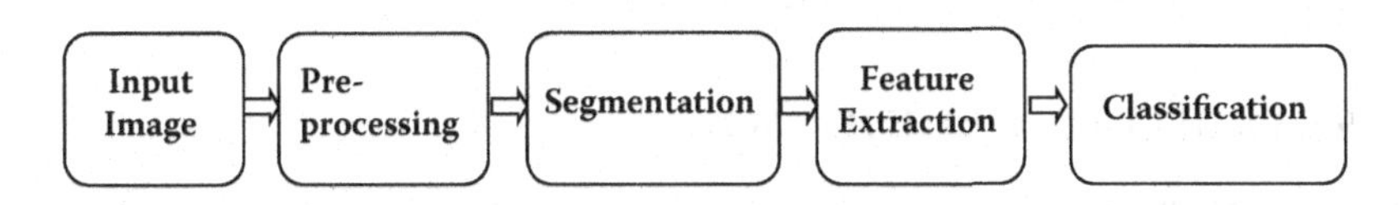

FIGURE 13.2 Basic Steps of Lung Tumor Detection.

The fundamental elements of numerical morphologies are the capacity to portray and recognize symmetrical structures in pictures quantitatively. But geometric structures can distinguish sizes or shapes portrayals, 3D connections amongst objects and topological property of articles. In view of its capacity in breaking down geometric highlights, scientific morphology become a significant guide in picture investigation application. Assortment of morphological application incorporates picture upgrade, picture division, picture rebuilding, edge identification, surface examination, highlight age, skeletonization, shape investigation, picture pressure, include recognition, space-time sifting, clamor concealment, design investigation, molecule extraction, imperfection investigation, little locale disposal, opening filling, line diminishing, layout coordinating, and shape smoothing [17].

When contrasted with a straight customary sign/picture preparing frameworks numerical morphology, varies in its nonlinear nature, since it doesn't fulfill an added substance superposition property. The primary issue with direct channels is that they are not planned from a basic perspective, so the resultant picture is an obscured one. Numerical morphology takes care of the above issue with the assistance of nonlinear super situation of pictures utilizing its association (maximal) and crossing point (minimal) activities. In morphological frameworks signals or pictures are seen as sets rather than capacities. In this way, the association/convergence activity is considered rather than expansion/deduction, individually [18].

13.4 OBJECTIVES OF STUDY

The significant constraints of previously mentioned examinations are their high pace of FP per check. Lower differentiate contrast between subsolid injuries and the encompassing lung parenchyma further hampers the division and volumetric evaluation of these knobs. Following are the targets of the investigation [19]:

i. The objective behind the work done in this examination to create procedures for the extraction of shallow and volumetric highlights in three dimensional advanced pictures utilizing morphological strategies.
ii. To prepare the framework for introduction of an exact and reliable framework for early location of lung knobs.
iii. To identify diverse trademark design for shape and size of lung knobs.
iv. Design and advancement of lung division dependent on grouping approach.
v. Effective knob extraction technique dependent on CNN.
vi. Implementation of knob discovery approach dependent on segment examination and utilization of huge component.
vii. Efficient knob discovery framework as far as reality multifaceted nature.
viii. Detail investigation of the outcomes.

13.5 PROPOSED METHODOLOGY

When CNNs are used for enormous collections of information, which is really the prerequisite in order-based applications, more calculation is required. Figure 13.3

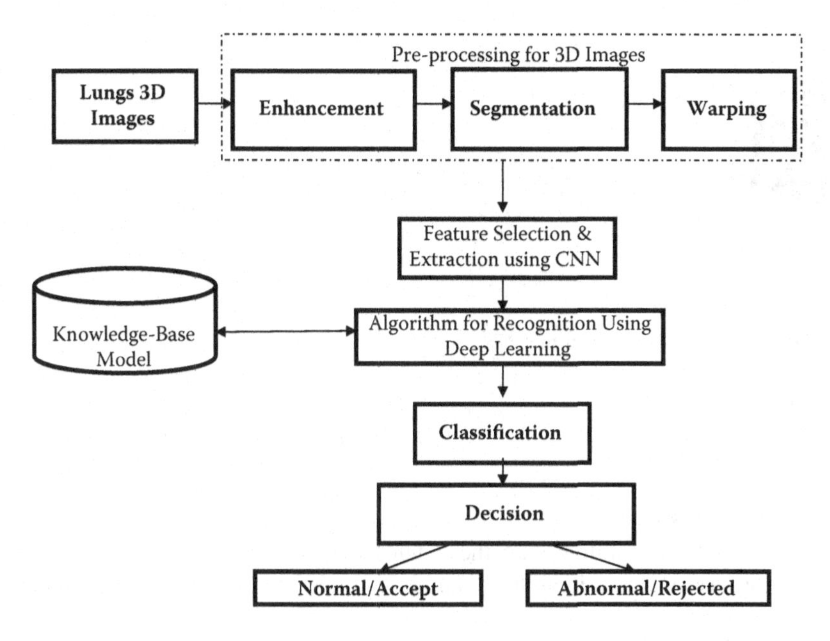

FIGURE 13.3 Workflow Diagram.

shows a run- of -the -mill engineering of the profound neural system [20]. In the proposed method, CNN is used for the classification purpose, which is represented in Figure 13.4 and Figure 13.5.

13.5.1 Evaluation Results for Medical Image Handling

13.5.1.1 False Positive Rate (FPR)

The level of situations where a picture was sectioned to the shape, however in certainty it didn't.

$$FPR = \frac{FP}{FP + TN}$$

13.5.1.2 False Negative Rate (FNR)

The level of situations where a picture was sectioned to the shape, however in certainty it did.

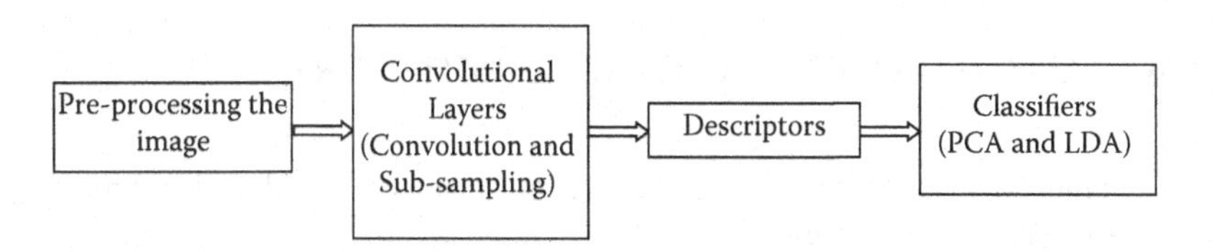

FIGURE 13.4 Block Diagram of a Typical CNN Architecture.

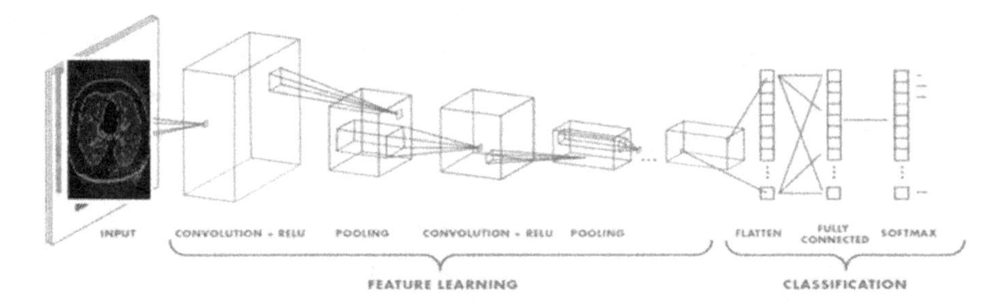

FIGURE 13.5 Block Diagram of CNN.

$$FNR = \frac{FN}{FN + TP}$$

13.5.1.3 Sensitivity

Proportions of affectabilities are the extents of real positivity which are appropriately observed. And it identifies with limits of tests to identify positive outcome.

$$Sensitivity = \frac{Number\ of\ true\ positives}{Number\ of\ true\ positives\ +\ Number\ of\ false\ negatives} \times 100$$

13.5.1.4 Specificity

Proportions of the particularities are extent of negativity which are appropriately observes. And it identifies with the limits of tests to identify negative outcome.

$$Specificity = \frac{Number\ of\ true\ negatives}{Number\ of\ true\ negatives\ +\ Number\ of\ false\ positives} \times 100$$

13.5.1.5 Accuracy

The weighted level of posture variety pictures is accurately characterized by the estimation exactness. It is spoken to like,

$$Accuracy = \frac{TP + TN}{TP + FP + TN + FN} \times 100$$

13.6 EXPECTED OUTCOME OF RESEARCH WORK

- Complexity of the created calculation must be contrasted with reference to time, space, and progress.
- Comparative investigation of created calculations with existing techniques.

13.7 CONCLUSION AND FUTURE WORK

In this paper, a model is proposed for the diagnosis of lung cancer using convolution neural network. The proposed method consists of preprocessing technique, segmentation of tumor from the given image and finally the classification of a detected tumor as cancerous or not. The outcomes were approved beside the clarified ground reality provided by four master radiologists. The proposed investigation fundamentally lessens the quantity of bogus positives (FPs) in the distinguished knob applicants. This strategy shows a general exactness of over 80% at a diminished FPs/examine pace of 0.50. The proposed framework demonstrated an improvement in lung knob location precision and can be usable in clinical settings. In future, a hybrid system can be designed such as by combining the neural network with fuzzy logic system which may improve the classification accuracy.

REFERENCES

1. Patil, D. S. and Kuchanur, M. (2012). Lung cancer classification using image processing. International Journal of Engineering and Innovative Technology (IJEIT). 2(2), pp. 55–62.
2. Chaudhary A. and Singh, S. S. (2012). Lung cancer identification on CT images by using image processing. IEEE International Conference on Computing Sciences (ICCS). pp. 142–146.
3. Hadavi, N., Nordin, M., Shojaeipour A. (2014). Lung cancer diagnosis using CT-scan images based on cellular learning automata. In the proceedings of IEEE International Conference on Computer and Information Sciences (ICCOINS). pp. 1–5.
4. Camarlinghi, N., Gori, I., Retico, A., Bellotti, R., Bosco, P., Cerello, P. Gargano, G. E. L. Torres, R. Megna, M. Peccarisi et al. (2012). Combination of computer-aided detection algorithms for automatic lung nodule identification. International Journal of Computer Assisted Radiology and Surgery. 7(3), pp. 455–464.
5. A. A. Abdullah and S. M. Shaharum(2012), "Lung cancer cell classification method using artificial neural network," Information Engineering Letters. 2(1), pp. 49–59.
6. Kuruvilla, J. and Gunavathi, K. (2014). Lung cancer classification using neural networks for CT images. Computer Methods and Programs in Biomedicine. 113(1), pp. 202–209.
7. Bellotti, R., De Carlo, F. Gargano, G., Tangaro, S. Cascio, D., Catanzariti, E., P. Cerello, S. C. Cheran, P. Delogu, I. De Mitri et al. (2017). A cad system for nodule detection in low-dose lung cts based on region growing and a new active contour model. Medical Physics. 34(12), pp. 4901–4910.
8. Hayashibe, R. (1996). Automatic lung cancer detection from X-ray images obtained through yearly serial mass survey. IEEE International Conference on Image Processing. DOI: 10.1109/ICIP.1996.559503.
9. Kanazawa, K. M., and Niki N. (1996). Computer aided diagnosis system for lung cancer based on helical CT images. 13th IEEE International Conference on Pattern Recognition. DOI: 10.1109/ICPR.1996.546974.
10. Salman, N. (2006). Image segmentation based on watershed and edge detection techniques. The International Arab Journal of Information Technology. 3(2), pp. 104–110.
11. Kumar, A. Kumar, P. (2006). A New Framework for Color Image Segmentation Using Watershed Algorithm. Computer Engineering and Intelligent Systems. 2(3), pp. 41–46.
12. Mori, K., Kitasaka, T., Hagesawa, J. I., Toriwaki, J. I. et al. (1996). A method for extraction of bronchus regions from 3D Chest X-ray CT images by analyzing structural features of the bronchus. In the 13th International Conference on Pattern Recognition. pp. 69–77, Vol 2.

13. Dwivedi, S. A., Borse, R. P., Yametkar, A. M. (2014). Lung cancer detection and classification by using machine learning and multinomial Bayesian. IOSR Journal of Electronics and Communication. 9(1), pp. 69–75.
14. WafaaAlawaa, Mahammad Nassef, Amr Badr (2017). Lung cancer detection and classification with 3D convolutional neural network (3D-CNN). International Journal of Advanced Computer and Application. 8(8), pp. 409–417.
15. Armato, S. G., McLenman, G., Clarke, L. P. (2011). National Cancer Institute, Lung Image Database Consortium (LIDC) and Image Database Resource Initiative (IDRI). 38(2), pp. 915–931. https://www.ncbi.nlm.nih.gov/pmc/articles/PMC3041807/.
16. Rohit Raja, Tilendra Shishir Sinha, Ravi Prakash Dubey (2015). Recognition of human-face from side-view using progressive switching pattern and soft-computing technique, Association for the Advancement of Modelling and Simulation Techniques in Enterprises, Advance B. 58(1), pp. 14–34, ISSN: -1240-4543.
17. A. C. Bhensle and Rohit Raja (2014), An efficient face recognition using PCA and Euclidean Distance classification, International Journal of Computer Science and Mobile Computing, 3(6), pp. 407–413. ISSN: 2320–088X.
18. Raja, R., Kumar, S. and Mahmood, M.R. (2020), Color Object Detection Based Image Retrieval Using ROI Segmentation with Multi-Feature Method. Wireless Personal Communications, pp. 1-24.
19. Rohit Raja, Tilendra Shishir Sinha, Raj Kumar Patra and Shrikant Tiwari (2018), Physiological trait based biometrical authentication of human-face using LGXP and ANN Techniques, International Journal of Information and Computer Security. 10(2/3), pp. 303–320.
20. Shraddha Shukla and Rohit Raja (2016), Digital image fusion using adaptive neuro-fuzzy inference system, International Journal of New Technology and Research (IJNTR). 2(5), pp. 101–104, ISSN:-2454-4116.

Index

Note: *Italicized* page numbers refer to figures, **bold** page numbers refer to tables

D

N

O

P

Q

R

S

T

U

V

W

Printed in the United States
By Bookmasters